Penguin Health

Living with Asthma and Hay Fever

After National Service in the Rifle Brigade, John
Donaldson read PPE at Christ Church, Oxford, and has
made his career in industry including, at one time, the
pharmaceutical industry. A lay member of the Executive
and Medical Advisory Committees of the Asthma Society
and Friends of the Asthma Research Council, he writes
regularly for *Asthma News* both on the work of the
Society and on the research carried out under grants
awarded by the Council.

JOHN DONALDSON

LIVING WITH ASTHMA AND HAY FEVER

Penguin Books

PENGUIN BOOKS

Published by the Penguin Group
27 Wrights Lane, London W8 5TZ, England
Viking Penguin Inc., 40 West 23rd Street, New York, New York 10010, USA
Penguin Books Australia Ltd, Ringwood, Victoria, Australia
Penguin Books Canada Ltd, 2801 John Street, Markham, Ontario, Canada L3R 1B4
Penguin Books (NZ) Ltd, 182–190 Wairau Road, Auckland 10, New Zealand

Penguin Books Ltd, Registered Offices: Harmondsworth, Middlesex, England

First published 1989
10 9 8 7 6 5 4 3 2

Filmset in Monophoto Sabon

Made and printed in Great Britain by
Richard Clay Ltd, Bungay, Suffolk

CONTENTS

12
THE QUESTIONS PEOPLE ASK –
AND WHERE TO FIND THE ANSWERS 197

APPENDICES:

FOREWORD

Nowadays the media are full of the marvels of modern medicine and greet even small discoveries as 'breakthroughs' so that it almost seems strange that anyone is ever ill. It is indeed true that serious illnesses which used to kill many thousands of people every year, such as smallpox, typhoid, cholera, pneumonia and tuberculosis, have been conquered by hygiene, vaccination and antibiotics. But several common ailments remain which, although not yet prevented or cured, can be controlled by powerful remedies discovered by medical science. These, however, only succeed if doctors and patients collaborate closely in their use. Old-fashioned 'doctor's orders' are of little use here. Patients have to learn about their illnesses and understand how their medicines act if they are to be effective.

Asthma and hay fever are typical examples of this situation. Modern treatments are now so powerful that the distressing and occasionally dangerous narrowing of the air tubes in the lungs, which causes difficult breathing, can be overcome by their use in all but a few especially difficult cases. And yet many patients remain disabled by asthma and the number of deaths it causes each year continues to rise.

There seem to be two main reasons for this sorry state of affairs. One is that many doctors, as students, were not taught how to spot asthma and haven't yet learnt about the new methods of treatment. The other is that some people with asthma seem almost to deny their illness, resent their dependence on health professionals and do not or will not take the trouble to learn about the nature of their asthma and its treatment. Moreover, few doctors are really good at teaching patients or can give time to it.

This is where a book like this one can be so useful. It is written by someone who has had to cope with severe asthma since he was a boy but has, at meetings of branches of the Asthma

Society, not only learnt how to keep his own asthma at bay but also has gone on to acquire a full understanding of the intricate and microscopic reactions in the lungs which cause asthma and how modern medicines can act to stop or reverse them.

If you have asthma, just learning all these details will not by itself ensure that you will manage to control it better. To do that, you have to decide (a) to understand your symptoms, (b) to see whether any of your present ways need changing, and (c) to follow any of the useful suggestions which you will find in these pages and which fit your particular sort of asthma or hay fever. The test of your success will be if you do as John Donaldson has done and have fewer attacks, less wheezing and greater physical activity; and studying this book will have been well worth the effort; if you have severe asthma it may even save your life.

Charles Fletcher, C.B.E., M.D., F.R.C.P., F.F.C.M.

PREFACE

Let us imagine that it is a beautiful day in early summer. You decide to take a stroll in the countryside. The birds are singing and you rejoice in the sight and smell of the flowers and the rich smell of newly mown hay; it feels good to be alive. But your joy is short-lived: your eyes begin to itch and stream, sharp needles seem to be at work in your nostrils and you soon feel listless and lethargic. You have hay fever.

On the following day the barometer falls and the weather changes. Storm clouds gather and then there is a squall of rain. You begin to notice that your breathing has become difficult and your chest feels as though a band has been placed round it and is being tightened. You start to cough and splutter; you feel ill at ease and a little apprehensive. You have asthma.

Of these two illnesses it is asthma which is the more distressing. It is true that hay fever makes you miserable: you feel as though your head is about to explode and concentration is difficult. But hay fever does not affect your speech or your ability to move around. Very few have died as a result of an attack of hay fever.

Asthma, on the other hand, if not expertly treated can be a handicap which is at times severe. It may deprive you of sleep, prevent you from taking exercise and make it difficult for you to move around at home. Even in a mild form it may lessen your confidence and efficiency at work. If it is severe you will not even be able to get to work. If the attack worsens to the point where you have the greatest difficulty in taking breath, then asthma becomes dangerous and immediate medical help is needed. For these reasons, many more pages will be devoted to asthma than to hay fever, which is in any case much easier to control. Both illnesses, even in the mildest form, have to be taken seriously.

My viewpoint is that of an asthmatic who, at various times,

has received most of the treatments offered by orthodox medicine for asthma and hay fever of varying degrees of severity, and who is now well controlled by them for most, if not all, of the time. I have not had experience of 'alternative medicine', though I can recall that in childhood I was required to smoke gold-tipped Abyssinian cigarettes, inhale incense from a smouldering powder and receive short-wave radio signals directed to some obscure region of the brain – remedies which were not so much unorthodox (they were recommended by conventional doctors) as bizarre!

My aim in writing this book has been at every stage to introduce the problems encountered by asthmatics and their families and to draw on high authorities in my search for the answers. 'Happy is he who can understand the causes of things.'

Fulham
September 1988

ACKNOWLEDGEMENTS

The ideas which form the basis of this book have derived mainly from talks given to three West London branches of the Asthma Society by specialists in or near the London area. These have included Professors Peter Barnes, Tim Clark, Barry Kay and Tak Lee and Doctors Anne Cockcroft, John Collins, Robert Davies, Bill Frankland, Donald Lane, Neil Pride, Michael Rudolf, Philip Snashall, Michael Silverman, John Warner and Derek Williams. Special thanks are due to Professor Margaret Turner-Warwick for checking, at various times, notes made from her talks on the physiology of asthma.

Certain chapters have been checked by Dr Douglas Jenkinson, Dr Michael Silverman and Dr John Stark. The manuscript as a whole was looked over at an early stage by Dr John Rees, Senior Lecturer at Guy's Hospital. Help has also been received in various ways from Doctors James Christie, Christopher Corrigan, Ian Gregg, Bryan Lask, Mark Levy and David Walker. Insights into the role of the physiotherapist have been provided by Miss Gaskell of the Brompton Hospital and Mrs Elizabeth Bell. I have been greatly helped by Dr Robert Pearson and Mrs Greta Barnes, S.R.N., whose course for nurses I attended at the Asthma Society's Training Centre. Mr P. J. Cousins has explained the role of acupuncture and Dr Anita Davies has provided insights into the principles of homeopathy.

Mothers of asthmatic children who have commented on parts of the text have included Marguerite Griffiths, Jenny Harries and Beryl Schirn. Felicity Hindson and Selina Thistleton-Smith have provided moral support from the same standpoint, and Eleanor Freeman commented on the manuscript from the point of view of the younger asthmatic.

With the kind permission of its Editor, Mr Hugh Faulkner, I have drawn material freely from *Asthma News*. A great deal of help has been received from the medical advisory departments of Messrs Allen & Hanburys, Astra Pharmaceuticals, Fisons Pharmaceuticals and 3M Riker. In this context I would like to thank Dr Gillian Pover, Mr Keith Watson, Dr Sarah Hemingway and Mr Michael O'Rourke.

Professional help has also been given by Mrs June Sykes, on welfare payments, by Miss Judith Steward, who carried out research into social attitudes towards asthma, and by Mrs Monica Robb, Secretary of the Asthma Society, who suggested that I should write the book. I am grateful to my Editor, Pamela Dix, for judicious pruning.

I would particularly like to thank Professor Charles Fletcher for writing the Foreword and checking the final text. In 1980 he started the Asthma Society with Dr Donald Lane, on the assumption that asthmatics and their families can do much to help themselves, an idea which is gaining ground with increasing momentum.

Note

Throughout this book, all doctors are referred to as 'he'. This is not because the author believes that all doctors are males, but only for simplicity's sake and to avoid constantly having to use the ugly 'he/she' format.

Chapter One

LIVING WITH ASTHMA

Introduction

It is surprising to asthmatics, who can feel rather isolated, to learn that asthma is a common illness which affects as many as one child in ten. It most often appears for the first time at between two and five years of age, disappears in the late teens or early twenties and then remains hidden until, in about five per cent of all adults, it reappears in later life. Up to the time of adolescence it is twice as common in boys as in girls; after this the girls are equally likely to have it. Asthma can start at any age, from early infancy to the eighties.

In childhood and adolescence, asthma is most commonly mild and the attacks occur after intervals during which there are no symptoms. In adults it is often a continuous illness which has to be treated all the time. In about a quarter of asthmatics the attacks are of moderate severity, increasing to very severe in about three per cent of cases.

Even mild asthma can be disturbing. It may take the form of coughing, or wheezing, or breathlessness, or all three combined. If the attacks persist, the family is likely to be as concerned as the patient, but at a loss to know how to help. It is fortunate that children, with their enormous vitality, are resilient and tend to forget, in between attacks, that they are at risk. But older people, with their chronic asthma, may find that it changes their whole way of life. It was sad to receive a letter from an elderly woman who wrote: 'I don't go out that much because the attacks can come on so quickly and people don't know how to help me.' Much depends on the quality of medical care.

The improvement in treatment

I am old enough to recall many strange remedies for asthma and also the disturbing side-effects from drugs such as adrenaline, ephedrine and isoprenaline. Nowadays the medicines are so effective and safe that most asthmatics, if properly treated, can live full and active lives. Asthmatic children can now participate to the full in games and sports and are as likely as other children to compete successfully in the school championships. Older people with severe asthma have to adjust their lives to the illness; but they can remain mobile and active even though the asthma is present all the time. Even when taken on a daily basis, the new medicines are safe in that the side-effects need not be lasting ones. It is not surprising that they have been described by cautious chest physicians, not given to exaggeration, as 'wonder drugs'.

For the first time prevention is possible. Until the early 1980s the medicines used to treat asthma were seen as primarily aimed at reversing an attack; they had only a small role to play in preventing it. In the last few years this attitude has changed dramatically; medicines are now available which can prevent attacks from taking place. The reasons for this are a combination of three factors: advances by the pharmaceutical industry, new insights into the way asthma develops, and the self-help idea, the acceptance by doctors that the patient has a large role to play in his or her own treatment.

One of the aims of the new treatments is to dampen down the 'twitchiness' of an asthmatic's airways, so that quite large challenges can be tolerated on a permanent basis. Two related ideas that are gaining ground are (a) that the patient can adjust the treatment to suit the circumstances, and (b) that he or she can anticipate challenges rather than simply react to them.

The medicines may be taken either on a routine basis, for short periods, or according to the severity of the attacks. This requires some knowledge on the part of the patient as well as a determination to keep healthy. By way of guidance, in the last few years there has been a spate of articles, leaflets and books dealing with asthma and allergies. Self-help groups have been formed and these have supplied news sheets and arranged talks by specialists up and down the country. Quite recently doctors in general practice have begun to set up special clinics which asthmatics are encouraged to attend for regular check-ups.

Asthma is often poorly controlled

In spite of the marvellous medicines and the help that is now available, asthma is still poorly controlled in many families. This is borne out by recent surveys and the too numerous admissions to hospitals. Asthma is still responsible for more schooldays lost than any other illness and is the cause of millions of pounds being lost through absence from work. Asthma is said to be the only illness in Western civilization, apart from AIDs, that is on the increase; all other illnesses are diminishing.

What is the reason for this state of affairs, which more than one specialist has described as 'lamentable'? One of the reasons is the simple one that, although asthma has been around for a long time, the remedies now used are of recent origin.

Myths and anxieties have gathered round the medicines, and this has led patients to approach them with extreme caution. In the 1950s and 1960s, when corticosteroids were first used in large daily doses to treat rheumatism, alarming side-effects were produced. They were widely reported in the popular press, especially facial swelling. Such doses are now rarely given when treating asthma, except over short periods. In the last few years there has been concern about anabolic steroids, used by some athletes to build muscles. These are never used to treat asthma.

The word 'drug' which, strictly speaking, can be applied to any ingredient used in the pharmacy has now taken on quite sinister overtones and brings to mind such problems as addiction and drug abuse. It happens that none of the medicines used to treat asthma is addictive; but some asthmatics prefer not to take 'drugs'; instead they have turned to alternative medicine, or they accept the orthodox treatment but stop the doses too soon. A more detached view of the remedies would lead to their being taken more effectively.

Myths have gathered round the illness itself, and these too can stand in the way of successful treatment. It is a widely held misconception that asthma is 'psychosomatic', a kind of nervous disorder; this view is not shared by chest physicians. Many children and some adults think it may be 'catching', even though it is in no way infectious. Some parents and not a few asthmatics believe that asthma is a kind of life-sentence which condemns the patient to a permanent state of physical inferiority. That this is far from being the case is proved by the fact that many world-class athletes, in a variety of sports and games, are asthmatic.

The role of the doctor

Patients who are critical of their doctors complain that either they do not listen to the asthmatic's problems or they do not take enough time explaining the treatments. Doctors are often the first to admit that this may be the case, but they cannot find the time that is needed.

Patients can become confused when a change of doctor brings a change of treatment, sometimes with disparaging remarks about what was given previously. They should bear in mind that the medicines now being used were introduced as recently as the 1970s; that the forms in which they are presented are constantly changing, and that doctors have had only a short time in which to find out the good and bad points of the medicines in an illness which is both complex and varied. What suits one patient does not suit another. Doctors build their experience on a trial-and-error basis; to some extent they are conditioned by what was preferred when they last received any training.

Doctors in their turn have a complaint to make about some of their patients. This is that an asthmatic can get used to his or her symptoms and as a result demands rather less from the treatments than they should deliver. Such a patient goes along too readily with the idea that asthma is the kind of illness you should learn to live with, and therefore you make the least fuss possible. After a time the asthmatic forgets what a normal airway feels like and adapts his or her life to suit the illness to an excessive degree.

Doctors are also aware that some patients angrily or fearfully reject the very notion that they have asthma and refuse to take a remedy, since to do so would confirm that they do indeed have asthma! As a result, some doctors when confronted with a wheezy chest avoid the word 'asthma' and use a label such as 'wheezy bronchitis' instead. This may be less alarming for this kind of patient but it can lead to the wrong medicines being used.

Another reason why asthma may be poorly controlled is that the attacks often arrive suddenly and without much warning: they are hard to predict and the triggers which provoke them are constantly changing. The result is that the medicines are not taken in time, or at the appropriate dosage level, or are switched off as soon as the symptoms fade, with the result that the wheeziness soon returns. Asthma varies from day to day in the severity of its attacks, and the dosage may need to be adjusted as soon as the first warning signs appear. All this calls for more education than is possible in a six-minute consultation. Asthmatics need to know why the medicines have been prescribed, how to judge their effectiveness and when to summon help.

What is asthma?

The word 'asthma' has come down to us from the Greeks and simply means 'to breathe hard'. Breathlessness, wheezing and coughing may all suggest the presence of asthma; but this is not exclusively the case, since they can be produced by other illnesses.

The chief and most distinctive characteristic of asthma is the variability of these symptoms. They are likely to vary as between day and night time, from one season to another, and according to the many triggers which can provoke the attacks. The attacks may be separated by long intervals of time, which can be counted in months or even years, or they may occur very frequently, typically on a seasonal basis. In chronic asthma the symptoms would be continuous, if they were not prevented by treatment.

Sometimes the attacks arrive without warning; at other times there are signs – such as listlessness and irritability, a disinclination to eat, and a kind of unease – that the air passages are at risk. Asthma has been compared to a river, slowly descending towards the sea until it meets a cliff or escarpment, and then it tumbles headlong downwards.

When they do occur, the attacks may last for only an hour or so and then clear of their own accord (for example, after exercise). Sometimes, however, they may persist – as often happens when triggered by a cold in the head or by an allergen such as pollen – and then they can go on for a day or two, or even for weeks.

What does it feel like?

It is impossible to convey to someone who has never had asthma what an attack feels like. In mild asthma there is a feeling of tightness in the chest, experienced particularly when breathing inwards; it is rather like trying to inflate a tyre with a foot-pump – you can feel the resistance in your breathing tubes. In severe asthma the shortage of breath is like being involved in the closing stages of a fast race, or like choking in a room full of smoke.

In young children the symptom may be a persistent cough, which carries on through the night and for night after night, until both parents and the child are exhausted. This is not, in spite of the nagging persistence of the cough, a dangerous form of the illness.

It often happens that asthma is worse at night, for reasons which are not yet fully understood. Loss of sleep leads to tiredness and irritability during the following day. The asthmatic is understandably reluctant to summon help at night time, and when he or she consults the doctor in the morning there may be no vestiges of the illness, or indeed signs of any illness. It is not surprising that asthmatics tend to play down symptoms which cannot be reproduced on demand.

Not one cause, but many

It is often not easy – or even possible – to decide what causes asthma in an individual. Asthmatics often think they can pinpoint the causes, but they may well be mistaken. In recent years it has been fashionable for the popular press to attribute asthma, hay fever and food illness mainly to 'allergens'. Asthmatics have been keen to undergo tests in order to discover what are their particular allergic triggers; these may include house dust and animal fur, pollens and mould spores. But there are many other triggers which are not allergens, for example breathing in cold or dry air, catching a cold, or being exposed to chemical fumes. It is possible to be asthmatic without showing any allergic reactions when tested. It is equally possible to be allergic to many substances and yet never present any sign of asthma.

At any given moment there are likely to be not just a few triggers but many, not only the pollens and the house dust but also chemical irritants such as cigarette smoke and fumes from the local power station. My house is close to the power station which provides electricity for the London Underground system, and I live in constant hope that the wind will not move round to the east! Even people's emotional responses can fire an attack: the sharp intake of air during laughter can upset those very sensitive airways. Exercise also puts asthmatics at risk. The triggers do not work in isolation but can reinforce one another: sometimes it is the allergen which primes the whole delicate mechanism and an irritant which provokes the immediate reaction.

Some asthmatics are very specific in their reaction. They wheeze only when they meet a cat, or eat shellfish, or sleep on a feather pillow. Such people can take avoiding action. For most asthmatics, however, the very air they breathe is a kind of mist in which there are many ingredients to which their exquisitely sensitive airways can respond.

Is asthma dangerous?

Deaths from asthma are rare. At the time of writing, there are in the United Kingdom about 2,000 deaths from asthma in a population of about two million asthmatics, that is, one in a thousand. Half of those who die are aged 35 or under.

It is generally accepted that two-thirds of the deaths could have been avoided, given the appropriate emergency treatment. Very few deaths occur in hospital; they take place mostly at home or when being rushed to the casualty ward. As a mother whose teenager died of asthma on the way to the hospital said:

> If only I had known that asthma could be fatal, my daughter might still be alive. No one had told me that a seemingly mild attack could escalate so quickly.

As the quotation suggests, a severe attack can happen suddenly and with little warning. A fatal attack generally occurs between two and five hours after the onset; it follows that any acute and severe attack of asthma should be taken very seriously.

Deaths are not caused by heart failure arising from a strain on the heart, as is commonly supposed, but are due to the sharp reduction in the supply of oxygen to all parts of the body, especially to the brain. This lack of oxygen is shown in a developing blueness of the tongue, lips and nails, and the next stage is a gradual loss of consciousness.

In the 1960s in many parts of the world there was a large increase in deaths from asthma; this statistic coincided with the introduction on to the marketplace of aerosol inhalers. Were they in some way responsible? It is now believed that they was not the cause; what probably happened was that the new form of treatment made the patients feel immediately so much better that they went on to face challenges which overwhelmed them. In the 1970s the anti-inflammatory drugs were introduced: these dealt with an underlying cause of asthma, and the death rate declined.

Asthma deaths are again on the increase, and no one knows why. One theory is that because of the scares surrounding the 1960s' drugs and the use of steroids, some people are undertreating themselves. Again, it may be that the environment is becoming more hostile to asthmatics, who need to become correspondingly more skilful in managing their illness.

Pains in the chest

It is quite possible for a pain in the chest to accompany an attack of wheezing and an irregular heartbeat. This is not a heart attack, which is a term used to describe damage to a heart muscle resulting from a hardening of the arteries, and caused by high blood pressure and an unsuitable diet – but never directly by asthma. An attack of asthma does put an extra strain on the heart; the chest muscles have to work hard to pull air into the lungs and this extra work requires more oxygen. At the same time, less oxygen is getting into the blood from the breathing tubes, so the heart has to pump more blood round the body, and the heart rate goes up – just as it does when you take vigorous exercise. After the attack the heart soon slows down again and suffers no permanent damage. Even in old age, asthmatics manage to perform that necessary extra pumping of the blood without any ill effects. The chest pain may be due to the muscles of the chest having to work really hard, so they produce a sort of cramp. This disappears when the asthma attack subsides or as soon as you are able to relax and breathe more slowly and evenly.

People with asthma also inquire whether high altitudes are safe, for example when climbing or skiing. In general they find they feel better in the clean mountain air, and any wheeziness can soon be dispelled with an inhaler. Flying in a pressurized aircraft should cause no problems and may even make the breathing easier. If in doubt, ask your doctor.

Is asthma a modern illness?

It is tempting to suppose that asthma is a by-product of modern civilization: of polluted air, of chemicals in our food, of crowded travel and work places where germs are exchanged; or is due to urban stress and strain; full of hope, we believe that if we were able to go back to a more natural life, the symptoms would disappear.

This is not necessarily the case. As Dr Alex Sakula has reminded us, in a fascinating paper tracing the history of asthma, the ancient Egyptians referred to it in their writings on papyrus and treated the illness not only with the excrement of crocodiles – which we might reject – but also with an inhalation of herbs. The Chinese wrote about asthma as long ago as 1000 B.C., at which time they were using a cough linctus, made from a plant from which, in modern times, ephedrine has been extracted. In India, herbs were used 1,500 years ago (as they still are today); these were introduced into England in the present century by doctors who had served in the Indian Army. One of these imported herbs was Stramonium, which turned up in 'Potter's Asthma Cure'. This was a powder which, when set on fire, produced an incense; I was given it in childhood and can still recall its sharp aroma, rather like snuff. The ancient Greeks knew asthma well and thought it was brought about by the 'humours' being out of balance. Their treatment was an emetic together with dieting, or relaxation induced by sedatives, massage, hydrotherapy and auto-suggestion. They were aware that asthma is made worse by exercise and cold air, that it is highly variable and increases during the period of sleep.

Are remote rural people free from asthma?

It seems that asthma is quite rare in the rural communities of the Gambia, West Africa, but is common in neighbouring towns. When a southern Pacific island community had to be evacuated to a mainland city, the incidence of asthma in children doubled. Asthma has increased in Papua New Guinea since Westerners started to move in.

Various theories have been advanced as to why this may be so. One is that breast feeding is more common in remote rural areas than in urban communities. (This theory does not explain why, in England, children of West Indian and Caucasian families are equally likely to be atopic,* as measured by skin scratch tests, yet breast feeding is much more common among the West Indians.) Another theory is that when people move into the towns they eat more processed foods which contain additives of various kinds, and that the additives are to blame. This theory comes up against the fact that in modern Japan there is a low incidence of asthma. Studies at the Hammersmith Hospital in London have shown that children from Indian immigrant families are especially likely to develop allergies to certain Western-type drinks and foods: could this be due to the change in diet rather than to its nature?

---

* 'Atopic', literally 'out of place' (referring to the reaction rather than the trigger), is the clinical term for the allergic condition which can be responsible for asthma and hay fever.

Is asthma linked to class or environment?

Research suggests that, in the U.K. at least, all social classes are equally likely to produce asthmatic children; but there may be a link between the occurrence of asthma and where you live, especially if there is dampness and old or poor-quality housing. It is presumably easier to tolerate asthma if you have an office job rather than one which involves exposure to cold or chemically polluted air. I suspect that people in the lower income groups may tend to accept asthma as inevitable, while the better educated are keener to understand its causes and treatments.

'Why do I have asthma?'

This question is often asked, especially by children. The answer to it may be either quite simple or exceedingly complicated, depending on how deeply we try to penetrate into the mysteries of lung behaviour. It is quite possible to control the illness without bothering ourselves at all with physiology, and the question has no final answer; indeed it continues to puzzle the scientists who spend their lives trying to supply one.

An investigation into the question will at least help us to discover the answers to some other commonly raised questions: how the medicines are able to act on the airways by various routes and manage to avoid conflicting with one another; why more than one medicine may be needed; and the ingenious ways in which the drug companies have contrived to improve the safety of the medicines. Armed with some understanding of the causes of our illness, we can confront the widespread assumption that asthma is 'all in the mind'. We can also see how it may be possible to prevent attacks, as well as stopping them.

To understand why some people get asthma, it is necessary to start from a definition of what it is. The following definition, by Professor T. J. H. Clark, will set the scene for what follows:

Asthma is breathlessness caused by a spasm in the muscle of the airways which connect the mouth and throat to the lungs. When this muscle goes into spasm it narrows the airways, obstructs the flow of air, and prevents your lungs from efficiently passing oxygen to the bloodstream and removing carbon dioxide from it.

If asked to describe the lungs, many will answer, rather vaguely, that they are 'a kind of bellows'. We will have to do a little better than that; but first of all we should really start by considering the nose. Whatever its shape or beauty, and however great or small, it acts as a most efficient air filter, managing to take out about ninety-five per cent of the dust and germs from the air passing through it. It achieves this because the air enters the nasal passages through a narrow aperture and this becomes turbulent. The air is then thrown against **Mucus**, the sticky coating which lines all the nasal passages, including the sinuses. Minute hair-like protuberances called **Cilia** sweep away the old mucus, which is constantly replenished. The cilia are in constant motion, like a field of corn ruffled by a breeze. If we breathe through our mouths, this cleaning and conditioning do not take place. The mucus also makes the air moist and warm and so prepares it for the next stage of its journey.

The air then passes through holes in the back of the nose and enters the throat (the pharynx). This area also takes in food; it then divides into two separate tubes. One tube is the food pipe (oesophagus); this can be closed by a trap-door known as the epiglottis, which prevents us from inhaling food. The second tube is the windpipe (trachea); you can feel it if you place your thumb and forefinger just below your 'Adam's apple'. The trachea receives air from the throat and continues the cleaning process. It too is covered with sticky mucus, which is propelled upwards and outwards by the cilia, so we can either cough up the dirt and germs that get past the defences in our nose or swallow them and so render them harmless.

The trachea is the gateway into the lungs. It divides into two passages; one leads to the left lung, the other to the right lung. These air passages are known as the **Main bronchi** (we will examine this last word again, in greater detail, when we look at the 'bronchodilators'). The bronchi then divide like the branches of a tree; they divide again and again, getting smaller and smaller, until they reach an internal diameter of about ten microns. This may be hard to visualize, but coincidentally it means

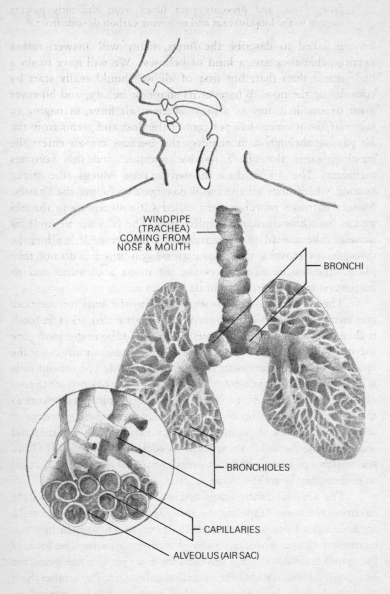

WINDPIPE
(TRACHEA)
COMING FROM
NOSE & MOUTH

BRONCHI

BRONCHIOLES

CAPILLARIES

ALVEOLUS (AIR SAC)

that the smallest bronchi have the same width as the thickness of a piece of cotton sewing thread. At this stage the bronchi are known as the **Bronchioles** – but it may be easier to refer to them simply as 'the tiniest airways'.

These very small passages lead to tiny air sacs called **Alveoli**, whose job is to transfer the oxygen out of the air that has been drawn in, into the bloodstream. At the same time they receive from the blood a waste gas, carbon dioxide, so that it can be passed back through the lungs when we breathe out. The bloodstream is connected to the air sacs through very tiny vessels called capillaries. The lungs themselves are like a most complex sponge. There are about three million air sacs; if you add up the internal diameter of all of them, the result will be about the same size as the dimensions of a tennis court. The lungs as a whole fill most of the space between our ribs, but they weigh only about 1.5 kilograms – clearly a system of extreme delicacy. It is also enormously efficient: even if we take quite small breaths, enough oxygen is absorbed through the air sacs to enable us to survive.

The oxygen passed into the bloodstream is delivered to all the tissues of the body. If the supply of oxygen is very much reduced, not only does the heart fail to function properly but many other organs are also affected, the most significant being the brain. In a severe asthma attack a gradual loss of consciousness is a rare but possible outcome.

Powerful muscles, lying between the ribs and directly under the lungs and known as the **Diaphragm**, cause the lungs to expand and contract. As the rib cage expands and the diaphragm contracts and pulls downwards, air is sucked into the lungs. Then the muscles relax and go into reverse to allow the lungs to return to their original size: this is the mechanism of expiration.

The activity of these lung muscles is controlled by a part of the brain known as the **Respiratory centre**. This adjusts the rate at which we breathe and also the amount of air drawn in at each breath. When we run for a bus or go for a brisk walk or become excited, we breathe faster and more deeply; this provides the extra oxygen needed by the heart, which has to pump the blood round the body at a rate which suits the activity. In sleep we need less oxygen, and the air machine relaxes to some extent – but of course we still carry on breathing.

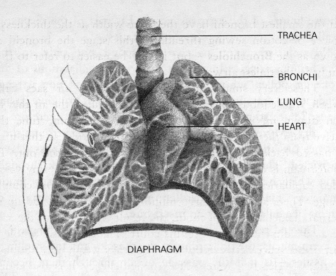

The respiratory centre adjusts the air intake all the time. It has to work out how much oxygen (and carbon dioxide) there is in the blood and also how much oxygen we need at each moment. This goes on about 30,000 times every twenty-four hours without any conscious control on our part; it is 'involuntary'. For most of the time we take breathing for granted; we become aware of it only when it becomes laboured: when we climb a mountain, or catch a whiff of smoke from a fire, or suffer an attack of asthma. In these situations we can usually intervene and control the lung muscles: we can decide to breathe more slowly or more deeply. But in a very severe attack of asthma we lose this control. Breathing becomes rapid, shallow and automatic, however hard we may try to breathe more deeply. We may even have so little breath that we cannot speak.

What happens when we wheeze?

Anyone exposed to strong fumes, to a thick cloud of dust or to the smoke from a bonfire is likely to cough and choke and bring up mucus. The mucus, or phlegm, is there to protect the delicate linings of the air passages and is part of the mechanism we all have for removing offending particles.

People who are asthmatic respond not only to these overwhelming triggers but also to very small inhalations of dust, smoke or pollen which would not affect their non-asthmatic friends in any way. It is not simply a question of bringing up more mucus. Some asthmatics produce very little and are therefore said to be 'dry'. More significantly, the muscles which surround the air passages in the lungs react by tightening, so passages are constricted. The effect is rather like trying to drink through a straw which has collapsed. In addition, the tissues surrounding the airways may become swollen, in much the same way as our skin may be inflamed after an insect bite.

The end result of all these actions on our breathing tubes – the extra mucus, the tightening of the muscles and the swelling of the tissues – is that the passage of air through them becomes difficult. This results in wheeziness, and since the action is likely to take place in many parts of the lungs at the same time, a difficulty in breathing.

A closer look at the air passages

Wheeziness is like the pursing of the lips when we whistle or allowing air to escape through the neck of an inflated balloon. These analogies are quite helpful, but they may lead us to think of the breathing tubes as if they were like the inner tube of a bicycle tyre or a collapsible plastic toothpaste tube, imagining something resembling a single layer of tough rubber or plastic. What the scientist sees, when he studies a section from one of the air passages through a powerful microscope, is much more complicated:

- on the outside, a band of muscle
- then a layer of connective tissue
- then 'mucosa' (glands which secrete sticky mucus)
- then an inner lining (epithelium)
- attached to this the cilia

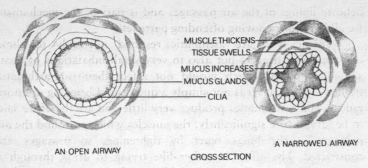

MUSCLE THICKENS
TISSUE SWELLS
MUCUS INCREASES
MUCUS GLANDS
CILIA

AN OPEN AIRWAY
CROSS SECTION
A NARROWED AIRWAY

Fig 3

This diagram will enable us to look at the components of asthma in a little more detail.

MUSCLE SPASM

In most attacks of asthma, the band of muscle which surrounds the air passages thickens, narrowing the aperture. This action is 'involuntary': we cannot control it consciously in the way that we can control the muscles in our hands. To use a medical term, there is **Bronchospasm**. This can take place very rapidly, in both the large and the small air passages; but it rarely occurs in all the passages at the same time, so we are able to continue drawing adequate amounts of air.

The sound of wheezing is caused by spasm or a thickening in *large* air passages, such as the windpipe. (Movement of air through the smallest airways is much slower and, even when they are narrowed, this does not cause wheeziness.)

It is not understood why the muscles go into spasm, since this does not appear to serve any useful function. A similar tightening occurs when we cough, in order to increase the rate of air flow needed to expel the mucus. But this is needed only in the larger breathing tubes, whereas spasm can affect the tiny ones as well.

INFLAMMATION

This is the way our bodies respond to an attack by an invader. For example, if we cut a finger and there is infection, white blood cells arrive on the scene and overwhelm the germs: the skin tissue becomes reddened ('inflamed') and swollen. In an asthma attack the same kind of reaction takes place, inappropriately, in the connective tissues of the airways. White blood cells invade the tissue; the vascular cells, which are normally half empty, fill up with blood; and as a result the tissue swells and further narrows the airway. This can take place very rapidly.

A glance at Figure 3 will show at once that a quite small increase in the thickness of the airway muscle will produce a much bigger reduction in the size of the airway when the tissue becomes inflamed. Even in mild asthma there is a certain amount of inflammation, and this is why scientists are spending so much time studying ways to prevent it.

STICKY MUCUS

Our story is not complete for there is yet another factor. In many attacks of asthma, the mucosal glands in the air passages secrete mucus in much larger quantities than usual, and it is sticky. This mucus is not necessarily infected (although this is a possibility) but it may be mixed with the debris of dead cells, so that when the airway muscles go into spasm they can squeeze the mucus into a thin sticky rope. This is hard to dislodge, especially as none of the drugs used in asthma has much effect in thinning mucus. These rope-like plugs are less common nowadays, possibly because there is less smoke in the atmosphere.

LEAKY LININGS

Even in mild asthma the inner lining of the airways, the **Epithelium**, can become leaky and allow irritants to penetrate to the nerve endings which lie just beneath it. These nerves can send a signal to the bronchial muscle and cause it to go into spasm. In a severe asthma attack the epithelial linings break down, adding to the debris inside the airway and knocking out the cilia which are attempting to clear it.

The way a severe attack develops if unchecked with medicines is shown in the form of a diagram on page 144 in Chapter Six. Very few attacks take the full course shown in this diagram, and almost all can be controlled at various stages. However, it may be asked how the body manages to take in enough oxygen when an attack is under way. Part of the answer has already been given: the tubes are affected patchily. It should also be borne in mind that when we breathe normally we use only half the capacity of the lungs, taking in about one and a half litres of air. By taking a deep breath inwards we can double the capacity to three litres.

Asthmatics learn to compensate for their illness by inflating their rib cages and lowering their diaphragms; when they cannot breathe more deeply, they breathe faster, in proportion to the severity of the attack. Furthermore, asthmatics learn to reduce the volume required by resting. When we walk we take twice the volume of air compared with that which is needed when we are sitting down.

Is there any permanent damage?

The reader may be assured that in asthma – unless it has been severe and poorly controlled over a long period – there is no permanent damage to the lungs, that is to say, to the alveoli or breathing sacs: they are not affected by asthma. (This is in direct contrast to chronic bronchitis due to heavy smoking, where there is lung damage and impaired capacity. Emphysema is a related condition, also caused largely by smoking, in which the lungs gradually lose their resilience.)

Just as damaged skin tissue is rapidly replaced when we suffer an abrasion, so the epithelial cells and cilia too are quickly replaced. However, the aim will always be to try to control the attack before cells start to break down.

Allergy as a cause of asthma

So far we have looked at what happens in asthma but not at the triggers which can initiate an attack. Chief among these, at least in childhood asthma, are the 'allergens'. This word is sometimes used to embrace all the triggers which can be inhaled, but here we restrict its use to those which are of plant or animal origin and show up on skin scratch tests.

Allergy has been defined as a state 'in which you are abnormally sensitive to a particular substance'. This abnormal sensitivity can make you feel itchy, it can make your eyes water, or you can feel sick – or it may make you wheezy. The symptoms may occur in the skin (causing eczema or urticaria), in the bowels (leading to diarrhoea), in the nose (causing hay fever) or in the lungs (producing asthma).

As we shall see in the next chapter, the allergens, in the narrow sense, are referred to as 'specific' triggers. They are mostly proteins and they may arise from dead as well as from live animals or plants; from textiles as well as from cats. Common allergens include:

- the house dust mite (which likes especially to live in mattresses and blankets)

- pollen (which also causes hay fever and makes the asthma worse in the summer)

- dander and saliva (especially from cats, dogs and horses)

- foods (especially milk, eggs and yeast in young children)

- fabrics (especially wool)

Allergens are not the only 'triggers' which can cause asthma. There are many irritants which are 'non-specific' and can provoke asthma in sensitive airways. These include: airborne pollutants, such as cigarette smoke and car exhaust fumes; chemicals in food and drink; virus infections; the action of cold and dry air on sensitive airways, especially during exercise; and 'over-breathing', due to emotion expressed in tears or laughter.

In infants the most common cause of asthma is not allergy but virus infection (though allergy may be added as a second trigger). In children up to the teenage years, house dust mite plays an important role, then pollens take over as the main trigger. In adults the most common causes are not allergens but infections and other irritants. The above listing is of course a simplification: both allergens and non-specific irritants are likely to be present in some degree when there is asthma.

Pollen grains and mast cells

To understand more fully the allergic response in asthma, let us take the example of a pollen grain. In early summer I sniff a

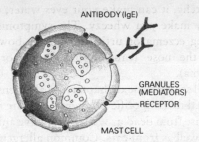

Fig 4a

cloud of pollen. Most of it is filtered out by the nose, but a small proportion manages to enter the larger breathing tubes in the lungs. The lining of these tubes is thin, and if it is leaky the pollen grain will be able to penetrate the airway tissues. Antibodies are then summoned to the scene, and in atopic people these arrive in large numbers.

What happens next will be more easily understood if we refer to Figures 4 a–d. The antibodies lock into **Mast cells** which are present in the tissues of the airways. These are now primed so that, when the next invasion of pollen takes place, the antibodies trigger the mast cells, which then release chemicals known as 'mediators' because they initiate a number of responses.

THE MAST CELL RESPONDS TO POLLEN

1 The mast cells are widely distributed, but here we are concerned with those which make their home in the linings of the breathing tubes. Each tiny mast cell has up to half a million receptors ready to attract IgE* **Antibodies** from the blood supply. Each antibody is specific to a particular kind of trigger, or **Antigen** (be it a pollen grain, animal dander or the faeces of the house dust mite).

2 As a result of an initial response to an intake of an antigen (such as pollen), into the lungs, the IgE 'pitchforks' lock into an appropriate receptor on the mast cell. The mechanism is now 'primed', but as yet no symptoms are experienced.

---

* IgE (Immunoglobulin Type E) is the chemical name for the antibodies.

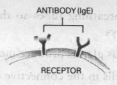

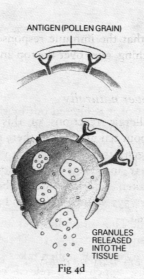

Fig 4d

3 A few hours, days or weeks later, there is another exposure to this same antigen (i.e. more pollen) and this now forms a bridge across two IgE pitchforks and the result is that the mast cell leaks or quickly releases its store of granules (chemical **Mediators** such as histamine, leukotriene, and prostaglandins).

The role of histamine

The way this procedure works can be illustrated by just one of the mediators which is released by the mast cell: histamine. (This name is already familiar if we have taken 'anti-histamine' drugs to relieve hay fever.) When it is released into the air passages and their underlying tissues, it can:

• Irritate the nerves which control the smooth muscle which

surrounds the larger breathing tubes so that the muscle thickens and narrows the airways

- make the mucus glands produce more mucus
- cause blood cells in the connective tissue to fill with blood and swell

The result is that the immune response to pollen, far from protecting our breathing, goes over the top and impedes it.

We may recover naturally

With most allergic reactions of this kind the wheezing reaches a peak in about ten minutes. If there is no further invasion of the allergen (antigen), then the wheezing will decline in an hour or so and disappear in a few hours more, even though no medicine has been taken. This response can be tested by measuring the calibre of the airways before, during and after a challenge by a single inhaled allergen.

But the recovery may be delayed

It is usually difficult to avoid further contact with the allergen. The pollen grains reappear in the atmosphere, so the challenge is repeated. This time, it is not only histamine which is released from the mast cells but also leukotrienes and prostaglandins. These not only cause the smooth muscle to thicken, they also attract to the scene white blood cells, including eosinophils and neutrophils which have their origin in the bone marrow. These white blood cells carry antibodies on their surface and can in turn be switched on by the invading pollen. Neutrophils add to the swelling of the connective tissue. Eosinophils do even more damage because they can diminish the thin lining (epithelium) which protects the airways from invading irritants.

It is the arrival of these white blood cells which produces the delayed or second-phase response. This is more severe than the original attack of wheeziness; it may take hours, days or even weeks to appear, and a corresponding length of time to disappear.

The second-phase response is harder to reverse with medicines; when it reaches a certain stage, it is the one that can become dangerous. It should be emphasized that, for most asthmatics, the attacks are mild and do not develop into this second phase. The aim of preventive medicine is to reduce the possibility of a severe attack taking place.

A closer look at the white blood cells

The picture we have just drawn is quite complicated, but it is not the whole story. It suggests that the mast cells initiate the asthmatic response. Using very sophisticated equipment, scientists have recently discovered that the mast cells are only accomplices: the real villain of the piece is to be found among the white blood cells. Earlier in this section we reminded ourselves that it is the white blood cells which come to our rescue when we cut a finger and need to repel the invading germs. One of these white cells has a special role to perform: its job is to alert all the other cells to the fact that they must act to overwhelm the intruders. It behaves rather like a policeman on the beat. This special kind of white blood cell, known as a lymphocyte, floats around in the blood stream in a dormant state until an invader, such as a virus infection, appears; it then becomes active and 'angry'. This reaction is beneficial when there is damage to body tissue; however, it is very undesirable when it takes place in the breathing tubes and leads to asthma: the policeman becomes the chief criminal!

In asthmatics, the lymphocyte is likely to go into action when it meets any kind of antigen, be it an allergen or a virus. It responds by secreting both antibodies and its own messengers, known as lymphokynes, whose task is to summon the other white blood cells to the scene. This is the response which is described as inflammatory; for example, when the eosinophils arrive they constrict the airways both by increasing the discharge of mucus, causing the airway muscles to thicken, and by damaging the linings of the airways. This makes the airways much more responsive to a wider range of irritants, including histamine released from the mast cells. It explains why a breakdown of the mast cells, which in normal people would not cause asthma, in asthmatics irritates the airways sufficiently to do so. It is the lymphocytes which make the airways 'twitchy'.

This explanation also helps us to understand why steroids are so effective in preventing asthma: there is a great deal of evidence that steroids can prevent lymphocytes from becoming active. It also explains why inhaled steroids have to be taken on a daily basis to prevent asthma; the lymphocytes are always present in the blood stream, ready to make their response to the antigens. Finally, it explains why it is so difficult to find a cure for asthma: it is the body's defence mechanism which is ultimately responsible for the attacks.

The scientists' task is made all the harder because all parts of the mechanism can influence one another through the system's very complicated circuitry. This means that, as soon as a scientist succeeds in blocking one pathway with the appropriate drug, another route is opened up by which the circuit can be switched on. It explains why drugs such as steroids, which intervene at an early stage in the cycle, are so valuable. Some of the pathways involved in the building of an asthma attack are shown diagrammatically in Appendix A on page 201, 'The secret life of cells'.

Non-allergic pathways

Asthma can be provoked by non-allergic triggers, for example by exercise, which increases the air intake and dries the breathing tubes so that various asthmatic responses are set in motion. Cold, dry air, and other kinds of irritants, can directly cause the mast cells to discharge their chemical mediators even though allergens and antibodies are not involved. The likelihood of this happening will be increased by a virus infection which damages the delicate protective lining of the air passages.

The role of the blood vessels

It may be asked by the inquiring reader how the white cells manage to get into the airway tissues. This matter is being studied intensively both by the basic scientists and by the drug companies: if the cells' entry could be blocked, then a cure for asthma would be found, as long as this action were confined to the lungs so that the whole immune system would not be put out of action.

As in other parts of the body, for example the skin, the airway tissues are fed by a rich supply of blood vessels, swiftly carrying along both red cells and white cells. The behaviour of the white cells is controlled by special chemical mediators, some of which when released into the bloodstream make the white cells sticky while others make the linings of the blood vessels sticky. This allows the white cells to attach themselves to the linings and then pass through them into the tissues, where they are able to set up the asthmatic response.

There is also another mechanism at work. The supply of blood to the tissues is governed by the constriction and dilatation of the muscles which surround the blood vessels. An increased volume of blood helps the white cells to accumulate and then leak into the tissues. This mechanism is partly controlled by a mediator (prostaglandin) but most durably by fragments of protein (CGRP) in the nerves supplied to the blood vessels. The action of CGRP is balanced by another mediator (Substance 'P') which can block it. By studying these intricate systems, scientists hope to be able to find a way of constricting the blood supply vessels in the lungs. It seems likely that exercise and emotion may affect these nerves and cause the blood vessels to dilate; since they may dilate to twice their normal volume, they also contribute to the 'inflammation' and explain the redness seen in airways which are constricted.

'Irreversible airway obstruction'

The end result of these complex responses is irreversible airway obstruction; this refers to all the ways in which the lumen (inner space) of the air passages can be made smaller:

- thickening of the smooth muscle wrapped round the airways

- inflammation of the connective tissue

- secretion of mucus into the airways

'Irreversible' does not imply that there is permanent damage but that the obstruction persists and requires medical treatment in order to restore breathing to normal. It also relates to the fact that the breathing tubes have become 'hyper-responsive' on a permanent basis so that, although the symptoms can be relieved, they are likely to appear again in the future in response to quite small challenges.

'Twitchy airways'

When I was young, doctors thought that spasm of the airway muscles was the main cause of asthma; their efforts were concentrated on reversing it with bronchodilators. In the 1960s it became clear that inflammation is also present in some degree. Later research has shown how the two may be linked. This gave rise to the concept of 'twitchy airways' or **Bronchial hyper-responsiveness** (B.H.R.). This can be illustrated with a simple diagram. An asthma attack will take place if

THE AIRWAYS ARE NOT VERY RESPONSIVE OR INFLAMED	...BUT...	THERE IS A VERY LARGE TRIGGER
THE AIRWAYS ARE VERY RESPONSIVE OR INFLAMED	...AND...	THERE IS QUITE A SMALL TRIGGER

Each of these circumstances can cause the airway muscles to thicken.

In non-asthmatic people, a trigger has to be very powerful and overwhelming to produce any narrowing in the airways – for example, a room full of dense smoke. In mild asthmatics, with airways either not at all or only slightly inflamed, it takes a sizeable trigger such as a heavy cold or a high pollen count or strenuous exercise to produce the symptoms of asthma. In people whose airways are more inflamed and 'hyper-responsive', it takes only a small trigger to cause the airway muscles to respond. A severe asthmatic may find, for example, that moving from a warm room to a cooler one can cause breathlessness.

In the next chapter we shall look at the triggers in some detail and find out whether there are any ways in which they can be reduced. Unfortunately, many of them are more or less outside our control. So our aim will also be to reduce the 'twitchiness' – in other words, to reverse the inflamed state of the airways. This will mean examining the various medical treatments that are now available.

Is allergy inherited?

We have looked at the various ways in which triggers can lead to asthma; in a later chapter we shall do the same for hay fever. But we have not really answered the question: 'Why do I get it and not my neighbour . . . surely it must be inherited?' Most asthmatics are able to point to some not too distant relative who has had an allergy of this kind. It remains a sober fact that about forty per cent of all allergy sufferers do not have a parent who is affected by allergy. This means that allergic parents do not always have allergic children – though there is a greater chance that they will do so if both parents are allergic.

What does seem to be inherited is the ability to make antibodies such as IgE in response to harmless as well as to harmful particles (to pollens as well as to germs), and to do so in large quantities. This is clearly a genetic defect. In an as yet unborn baby with atopic parents, higher levels of antibody can be detected in the blood in the umbilical cord than in 'normal' babies. What is needed to develop this inherited tendency is a sufficiently powerful initial challenge. Some people remain atopic without ever experiencing symptoms because this challenge has somehow been avoided, especially in early life when infants and toddlers are perfecting their immune systems.

Dr Julian Hopkin, a geneticist working in Oxford, is studying these matters both from family histories and by examining the genes themselves. It takes only a small change in the composition of one gene to produce a dramatic effect. It is now possible for the scientist to show where, along the very long string of DNA, the faulty bit can be found which is transmitted in atopic people, or in those with very responsive airways.

This does not mean that there will be a rush into genetic engineering – at least not in the next hundred years. We are not yet in a position to breed asthma out of the population. What *is* possible is practising some sensible 'marital engineering' on the lines described in Chapter Five, 'Questions that parents ask'.

It is also highly desirable, in the first three months of an infant's life, that the triggers described in the next chapter should be reduced as far as possible; this will lessen the risk of the child becoming sensitized to them. This observation derives from research in Sweden, where it has been shown that it is those babies who are born in the short, three-week birch-pollen season who are most likely to develop an allergy to birch pollen. Research under way at the Brompton Hospital, London, is confirming that this is true of all allergies when airborne.

Chapter Two

WHICH TRIGGERS CAUSE ASTHMA?

The nature of the problem

If you have managed to get through the previous chapter, you will be in no doubt that asthma is a complex illness which leads its sufferers to respond to very diverse triggers. Some of these are invisible and float in the air we all breathe; others arise from our lifestyle (what we do or eat, or from our work). Infection also puts asthmatics at risk.

TRIGGERS WHICH ARE:	TRIGGERS	TRIGGERS WHICH ARE:
'specific'	WHICH	'non-specific'
'atopic'	CAN	'non-allergic'
'allergic'	LEAD	'irritants'
	TO	
SEASONAL	THE	ALL YEAR ROUND
pollens	ASTHMATIC	exercise
moulds	RESPONSE	emotions
	OF	atmosphere
ALL YEAR ROUND	AIRWAY	pollution
house dust mite	OBSTRUCTION	chemicals
animal dander		food additives
certain foods		
		infection

There are three ways in which asthmatics can try to prevent their attacks:

- They can try to reduce exposure to the triggers
- They can be 'desensitized'
- They can take appropriate medicines

In this chapter we shall look at the triggers and ask about each: 'Is there any way in which we can avoid them?'

If you suffer from asthma mainly in the late spring and early summer, then it is probably due to an allergy to pollens. If the asthma persists into the autumn, then moulds are likely to be the triggers. If you have asthma all the year round, then it may be due additionally to an allergy to house dust mite, or to animals, or to food. On the other hand the trigger may be an irritant, such as a virus infection or air pollution. In this case the asthma is not due to allergy and is also likely to take place at all seasons.

Pollens, moulds and dust
The flowers that bloom . . .

. . . do so in order to attract insects to the pollen. The pollen grains they produce are heavy and sticky and do not travel very far in the spring and summer breezes. These are not the main cause of asthma unless they are brought into the house and are heavily scented. It is the lighter pollen grains (from certain trees, meadow grasses and weeds) that are mainly responsible for pollen asthma. When their season is due, they produce pollen in clouds which can be carried by the winds for hundreds of miles.

The pollen season lasts from April to August but reaches its peak in late June and early July. Leafy trees like the birch and plane pollinate in April and May, grasses from May to July and weeds (such as nettles and plantains) in July and August. In Scotland all this happens a week or two later. In North America, ragweed is a powerful source of wheezes.

Is it possible to escape a trigger which is everywhere in the atmosphere?

• Pollens rise up into the sky, high up into the clouds, during the morning. They descend again in the evening. So it is a good plan, during the pollen season, to open the windows only during the middle of the day. I have double-glazed the windows of my bedroom as an added precaution. Well-fitting outside doors are also advisable.

• Offices with air conditioning may keep out pollens. In the country, the car can be a temporary refuge from pollen, to bring an attack of asthma or hay fever under control.

• It has been suggested that you rinse your hair to rid it of pollen before you retire; pets, which can bring in pollen on their fur, should stay outside during the peak season.

• Choosing a suitable place for a holiday, to escape from pollens at home, is not all that easy: there is a problem of timing, because our season can vary by a couple of weeks, after a cool spring. It is a good plan to choose somewhere in the mountains or close to offshore breezes, though these do tend to reverse in the evening.

A mouldy business

If you feel wheezy during damp weather or just after the grass has been mown, or when you are standing near a stack of rotting compost, then you are probably allergic to moulds. If you feel better when the landscape is covered with snow, then this confirms it.

Moulds belong to the fungus family. They produce a pollen-like dust (millions of spores) which can travel around in the atmosphere. They lie dormant during the cold months, wake into life in the spring and remain active until well into the autumn. Very high levels are reached when the air is damp and during rainfall, especially at night. Their connection with allergy has been known for a long time, but very little work has been done on this: chest physicians are divided as to their importance as a cause of asthma.

Moulds like warm damp places, such as grass clippings, and the environment forests provide. The rich warm smell of newly ploughed fields comes from moulds. I moved to the seaward side of the New Forest in the hope of escaping from pollens: the asthma became worse. I read that in the Middle Ages the monks in nearby Beaulieu Abbey suffered badly from asthma – this may have been due to moulds in the surrounding forest.

They also flourish indoors, in damp basements, old wallpaper and upholstery, and even in modern foam furniture and rubber pillows when damp. Clothes in badly ventilated wardrobes can grow moulds. So can vegetable bins, pet litter and potted plants.

Modern ventilating systems grow moulds in the ducts and then spread spores round the offices, along with bacteria, pollen and air pollutants. It is difficult to escape from moulds or to eradicate them. You can try the following ways:

· Outside, in the garden you could replace the grass with a different form of ground cover, or use stone slabs or gravel instead, with plenty of shrubs to avoid the work involved in making extra flower borders. Better to buy mulches than to make compost.

· Inside the house, you may be brave enough to remove all the damp wallpaper and use emulsion paint instead. You could revert to the older style of light rugs on polished wooden floors instead of heavy carpets. You could also get rid of all the rejected but not discarded odds and ends which lie around in corners.

· All sources of dampness from outside should be removed, whether from a loose roof-tile, a blocked rainwater channel, or a pile of sand placed against an outside wall. Inside walls, if previously mildewed, should be treated with an anti-fungal solution, which can be obtained from your paint supplier.

· It is impossible to treat upholstery with any success and foam filling should be replaced from time to time (preferably with a type that does not constitute a major fire hazard).

· The old-fashioned routine of airing sheets and blankets outside could be revived, avoiding the pollen season. Clothes should be dry cleaned regularly.

· The rubbish bin and kitchen waste bins should also be kept clean. Borax is effective against moulds.

· The air inside the house, when the windows are shut, can be kept moving with electric fans. But this also means that it is essential to keep the floors free from dust: fans push it up into the breathing tubes. My worst ever attack arose in this way.

• Some people install dehumidifiers which switch on when the humidity rises above a certain level. Some humidity is needed to keep the nasal passages moist so that they can trap the invading particles.

• It is worth mentioning that certain foods and drinks which include yeasts may have to be avoided (see Chapter Seven, page 153).

Dust that builds on dust

One of the more imaginative English eccentrics, Mr Quentin Crisp, has pointed out that if you leave dust well alone it never rises above a certain thickness; much better not to disturb it, he believes. Unfortunately, this does not work because we stir it all the time.

What is dust? We tend to think of it as something that comes in from outside. This is only a small part of the story! Pollens from grass and weeds can be transferred from outside into the house. Arising from within, there are the skin scales shed by humans and the dander from pets; there are fragments of clothing and bedding and debris from upholstery; dust from the fireplace, dead insects, dead plant matter, food fragments and tobacco shreds.

The dust particles that trigger asthma attacks have to be small enough to penetrate the breathing tubes; to be 'allergic' they have to be derived from once living matter. The allergen that features at the top of most asthmatics' hit list is present in house dust: the **House dust mite**. It is 0.3 mm long and is invisible to the naked eye, even in large numbers. In its common form it is called rather grandly *Dermatophagoides pteronyssinus*; it has eight legs and, suitably enlarged, would win an Oscar in a horror movie.

House dust mites live on human skin scales and moulds wherever these are allowed to collect. They especially favour the folds in mattresses, feather pillows, thick carpets and old soft articles, such as toys. They can breed only at over fifty per cent relative humidity and they prefer a temperature of around 25°C. What manages to enter our airways is not the mite itself but its faecal pellets, which are light enough to become airborne and small enough to enter the airways.

What counter-measures can asthmatics take? In 1547 the then Archbishop of Scotland was visited by a famous physician, astrologer and philosopher, Geromo Cardano of Pavia. On learning that His Grace had severe asthma, the visitor recommended that the feather pillows be replaced by wooden ones. Nowadays we use instead pillows made from latex foam or stuffed with terylene. I personally take a small one with me when away from home.

We also have vacuum cleaners. Unfortunately the household models leak dust in all directions and the mites can migrate back into the furnishings. Remove the bag immediately after use and dispose of it in an outside bin. Cleaners designed for hospital use claim to collect ninety-nine per cent of the particles, and also to trap them within the filter (addresses are given at the back of the book). Unfortunately, even they cannot eliminate all the mites that live in the bedding and are likely to leave behind some of the mites' eggs, so that in a week or two their numbers are probably fully restored.

Physicians tend to be sceptical about these 'safety-first' operations and suggest that we rely on our medicines instead. I do not share this view. I know that I have much more difficulty in controlling my asthma when staying away from home, in hotels or private houses, and the worst attacks tend to take place at night in the bedroom. So I support Dr John Rees when he writes: 'regular cleaning of bedrooms and avoiding materials particularly likely to collect dust are worthwhile measures to keep down the allergenic load'. He also advises that while house dust mite desensitization may be of use in some children, it is not in adults.

We could avoid the mites altogether by removing to the French or Swiss Alps. Above 1,000 metres, the air is so dry that neither the mites nor the moulds on which they partly feed can survive. And this may help to explain why asthmatics often feel better after a holiday in those regions, at least for a time. Regrettably, this is not a practical long-term solution for most of us!

It may be asked why the mites cannot be eliminated with an

insecticide. In the past the answer has been that if it killed the mites it would also harm man. The solution may lie in using plant substances that we can tolerate, to kill the mites, and this is being investigated in Australia, using a miticide called 'Allersearch'. British allergists are sceptical about a house paint which comes from France with the (as yet) unproven claim that it will eliminate mites from bedrooms.

Until some way is found of eradicating the mites, we have to keep on with our cleaning measures, with the materials available to us, especially in the bedroom:

• We can encase the mattress in a heavy-duty polythene cover. (Some hospitals provide these.) They do tend to be slippery and liable to move out of place. Non-slip covers are now appearing on the market.

• Dunlopillo make latex-foam mattresses and have advised me that house dust mites cannot live in them. Such mattresses should be kept dry, to prevent moulds from appearing. A water bed is a possible alternative.

• Dr John Warner of the Brompton Hospital has suggested that an electric blanket would keep the temperature of the bedding above that which is suitable for mites breeding. Of course this would have no effect on mites in other parts of the bedroom, but it sounds worth trying.

• Mites prefer to live in natural fibres. Artificial fibres should be used for all bedding, carpet and curtains in the bedroom. They should also be used to fill the duvet cover, and there is no point in changing only one pillow on a bed provided for two! It is often a good idea to wash the bedding and pillows quite often, and our grandparents' insistence on hanging out bedclothes in bright sunlight, which kills mites, was a good one.

• If you have acquired a special vacuum cleaner and are determined to try to rid the mattress of mites, clean it every day for the first seven days, then regularly every week, with special attention to the buttons, which is where the mites like to live. If you vacuum in a dull light, the mites are likely to be closer to the surface. Avoid a padded fabric headboard – a perfect home for mites.

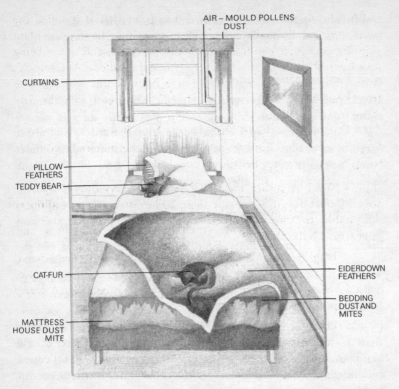

AIR – MOULD POLLENS
DUST

CURTAINS

PILLOW
FEATHERS

TEDDY BEAR

CAT-FUR

EIDERDOWN
FEATHERS

BEDDING
DUST AND
MITES

MATTRESS
HOUSE DUST
MITE

Fig 5

• Always use a damp duster, to avoid spreading the dust; clean under the bed and on top of door-frames, pictures and mouldings, as well as the more obvious places. Avoid upholstered furniture in the bedroom, and heavy curtains or Venetian blinds; roller blinds with a plastic finish are best. Wash light curtains and soft toys regularly in a machine.

• Mites thrive best at around seventy five per cent relative humidity; they cannot survive under fifty per cent humidity. People who install dehumidifiers have to be careful not to dry the air too much. Mites approve of central heating!

Dust removal is especially valuable in a situation in which a child becomes convinced that the dust is to blame for the asthma and this fear reinforces the constriction. If a really efficient cleaning method can be demonstrated, then the fear may disappear.

Pets and other animals

Allergists are severe about pets. They tell us that any animal, large or small, can sensitize a potentially allergic person and be the first cause of a child becoming asthmatic. This danger may not be evident for some time and can be compared to a time-bomb ticking away unnoticed. It is not the hair or fur of the animal that upsets an allergic person but the 'dander', or tiny flakes of skin, too small to be seen with the naked eye and light enough to become airborne along with the dust.

Cats are the commonest cause of allergic asthma and Persians and Siamese the worst offenders. With cats it is not the dander alone that causes the reaction but also the saliva, which dries on the skin and then becomes volatile. If the cat is around all the time, the allergic response may well be chronic. In extremely suggestible persons who have been conditioned by the response from a real cat, just the picture of a cat may be enough to start a wheeze. While cats lick themselves, dogs are also keen on licking any human whom they regard as an acceptable pack-leader, including children. This can cause urticaria, which is revealed as a rash.

Some physicians recognize that, where the asthma is mild, to remove a much-loved pet could cause undue suffering. In this case the animal should never be allowed into the bedroom. Others suggest a trial period of separation, to see if the symptoms improve. The house must be thoroughly cleaned at the start of the trial because particles of dander lie around for some time.

An animal does not have to be alive to cause wheeziness. Animal hair deposited in furnishings, furs on coats and, as we have seen, feathers in pillows can all cause allergies.

It is possible to use a skin prick test to confirm whether an animal is responsible. This is not always a reliable guide. Sensitivity may develop even though the test is negative; this is either because the solution used was not sufficiently specific or because the onset took place after the test. If the saliva of, say, a male Siamese is what is suspected, this is what should be used, in solution, in the test.

Replacing the pet dog or cat with a rabbit, gerbil, guinea pig or hamster is not a good idea. These animals are used by laboratory workers and a high proportion of technicians develop asthma as a result. This is partly caused by the urine, which becomes volatile and gives off its characteristic smell. It can take eighteen months for a child to be sensitized by them. Even tropical fish, which appear to be much too beautiful to harm anyone, may cause their owner to become sensitized – not to the fish themselves but to their food, such as ants' eggs. It seems that many Russians, who like to keep tropical fish in their apartments, suffer in this way.

It is rare for a child or an adult to be sensitive only to animals. However, this is not an argument for keeping them, since one allergy reinforces another. Remove one and you may reduce the impact of the rest.

It is well known that insects can cause allergic reactions through their stings, sometimes with severe consequences. The area round the sting may remain swollen for a day: this is no cause for alarm unless the swelling persists or the whole arm or leg swells. In that case you should see a doctor at once because you may be at risk of suffering 'anaphylactic' shock, which is like a very severe asthma attack and may lead to loss of consciousness and death. Incidentally, it is not the bite of a mosquito that causes the allergic reaction but the saliva which is injected along with the sting.

One man's meat is another man's poison

This is as true today as it was when first observed, in Roman times. Allergy to food receives a lot of attention nowadays, but chest physicians do not see it as a common cause of asthma. They also doubt whether avoiding action is sensible, except in those rather rare cases where the allergy can be traced to one particular type of food which can be eliminated and still leave the patient with a balanced diet. They take the view that it is simpler to rely on the medicines – especially since these have to be taken anyway, as asthma usually has many other triggers in addition to food.

That having been said, allergists are concerned that our complex factory-made foods may be contributing to the rising incidence of asthma, and they feel that serious attention should be paid to the substances added to ready-cooked foods. This topic will be discussed at greater length in Chapter Seven, when we shall have discovered what the medicines can do to relieve asthma (on page 59).

How can I tell what causes my allergies?

We have already seen how allergic persons develop antibodies against allergens such as pollen grains or house dust. When the allergen and the antibody meet, chemicals such as histamine are released into the sensitive tissues.

If histamine is released into the nostrils and eyelids, you start sneezing and itching (hay fever); if it is released into the breathing tubes, you become wheezy (asthma). If, on the other hand, it is released into the skin, an itchy swelling appears. This reaction is quite small and harmless, so doctors use it to find out what substances you are allergic to – or, rather, they used to do so, because the tests are not widely used nowadays.

This technique is called a skin prick test. The doctor drops a small extract of allergen suspended in water on to the skin of your forearm and then scratches it into the skin. By testing a range of different allergens in this way he can discover whether you are allergic (atopic) to various pollens (tree and grass), danders, house dust mite extract and moulds. If a small, reddish, itchy swelling appears then you are atopic to the substance in the extract. The test has serious limitations:

• It is possible to be atopic (positive results from the test) without ever having any symptoms of asthma or hay fever.

• It is possible to be atopic but to develop asthma from a cause which is not allergic, as for example a chemical at work or the intake of cold air.

• It is possible to be an asthma sufferer without being atopic to any of the substances scratched into the skin.

• Some people are atopic to one substance only: they are allergic only to cats or to certain foods such as shellfish. But most asthma sufferers are allergic to more than one substance, and many are atopic to all the extracts, though in different degrees as between one extract and another. In these latter cases, avoiding the substances is difficult, even impossible, and reliance on medical treatment alone would seem to be preferable.

A skin test can have some advantages. It can help the doctor confirm that the wheeziness is indeed an asthmatic response and is not due to some other lung disorder. It can help support the patient's own belief that a particular substance is responsible, and confound those who doubt this. And it can be a guide to treatment, for example, by suggesting to a horse-loving girl that she should take her medicine before setting out for the stables.

Why is desensitization less used?

We heard a great deal about desensitization in the days before the newer drugs were introduced, but don't so much nowadays. Why is this? The simple answer is that the newer medicines enable physicians to control asthma much more successfully so that the process is no longer necessary.

The aim of desensitization is to change the allergic response. By first giving the patient a series of extremely small doses of one or a couple of allergens, the immune system responds, but not excessively as in asthma. The doses are then increased gradually until the patient can tolerate the levels of allergen which would normally cause asthma.

First of all the doctor has to identify which allergen is to be used, with the help of the skin prick test just described. Treatment is started about six months before the season which causes most trouble, say the pollen season. The extract, in solution, is injected under the skin of the arm, at first every few days, then in increasing doses. Finally, a maintenance level is reached and the dose is repeated at this level, once a month.

The Ministry of Health has recently put out guidelines on desensitization. General practitioners may not now carry out the process and chest physicians may do so only within strict rules. The drawbacks are:

• There may be a violent, life-threatening response in a very small minority of patients, and the doctor has to have adrenaline at hand to be able to counteract this.

• Desensitization is valuable only in those cases where the patient has a very specific response to a narrow range of allergens (for example, reacts only to grass pollen or to cats). The injected substance has to be highly specific (for example, saliva from the appropriate breed of cat, or the right kind of fungal spores).

• In many cases the response from dummy injections has been shown to be no less beneficial, and this throws doubt on the effectiveness of the treatment.

The procedure is time-consuming and can be expensive for the patient. The majority of chest physicians (not trained as allergists) believe that a similar or better degree of control can be obtained by using an inhaler.

Exercise, emotions and chemicals

I have found that in middle age my asthma seems to respond much more readily to triggers which are not allergic in the strict sense of being due to atopy. Nowadays I tend to have less summer pollen asthma but I am much more sensitive to the 'non-specific' triggers, the ones that cannot be tested by skin scratch tests. This is a normal pattern. It occurs possibly because our immune reactions slow down when we grow older, so that on the one hand we become more vulnerable to infections and, on the other, less liable to immune responses to allergens.

Asthma due to exercise

Most asthmatics find that exercise is a trigger. In the young the response can usually be prevented with the appropriate medicine; in older, chronic asthmatics with severe asthma, this becomes more difficult to achieve.

A curious feature of asthma induced by exercise is that it gets worse after the exercise has finished, reaching a peak after a few minutes and then lasting for about half an hour, before it subsides. What happens is that at first exercise dilates the airways. Needing more air when we exercise, we take in a greater volume; this, even in summer, is relatively cool and dry compared with the warm moist air needed for passage through into the air sacs. Faced with such a large volume, the nasal passages are not able to condition it; the breathing tubes have to complete this task, so they lose water and the protection of the moist mucus blanket. The airways become 'leaky', the nerves which lie under the linings are triggered and mast cells start to release their chemical messengers so that inflammation of the air passages takes place.

Does this mean that asthmatics should give up taking exercise? The answer is an emphatic 'no', but they should adjust the exercise to what can be tolerated. There is no doubt that exercise taken in moderation can benefit everyone. It builds strong healthy children, provides a challenge for adolescents who are keen on sport, and in middle age helps keep heart disease at bay. In old age it helps avoid a tendency of muscles to sag. It is also good for asthmatics, helps them fight infections and improves the efficiency of their breathing so that they can perform better with fewer resources. Some doctors go further and claim that physically fit people are much better able to cope with mental stress than those who are unfit; they have a sense of well-being, are more confident and meet challenges more easily.

So asthmatics need to know how they can tolerate exercise. Some forms cause more wheeziness than others. It may be a matter of how much energy is needed. Running is worse than horse riding or cycling. Swimming causes very little wheeziness;

the body is supported and the warm moist atmosphere of a heated indoor pool is ideal for people with asthma.

How do you decide whether you stand in need of more exercise? You take a watch with a second hand and go to the foot of the stairs. Step on the bottom stair with one foot; bring the other up to it and then step down. Repeat the exercise 24 times within 60 seconds and then stop. After a further 60 seconds, take your pulse rate for a period of 15 seconds. You should count no more than 25 heartbeats for men and 28 for women under the age of forty-five. If your rate is above 20 you are unfit and would benefit from exercise.

How much exercise is needed? If you work out twice a week for 20–30 minutes vigorously enough to increase the breathing rate, this should be sufficient. But, you may object, even this modest amount may induce an attack of wheezing. This is an understandable worry – but there are various ways in which exercise can be tolerated by people whose asthma is normally affected by it.

• You can take the appropriate medicine, as explained in the next chapter. 'Intal' or a bronchodilator is taken before the exercise, and in addition it may be necessary to take a preventive medicine on a daily basis.

• Fitness can be acquired through a graduated swimming programme because of all exercises this is the least likely to provoke wheeze. The asthmatic can then progress to what we used to refer to at school as 'physical jerks' but which are now described less alarmingly as 'dry land' exercises. All the exercises should start gently with warming-up movements before becoming more strenuous. This enables the lungs to adapt gradually to the demands being imposed on them.

• Many athletes, including some Olympic gold medallists, have asthma; they find that, before a long distance run, a few short sharp sprints will release enough natural adrenaline to keep the breathing tubes relaxed. If exercise makes you short of breath, then an energetic sprint on the spot may do the same trick and prevent subsequent activity from provoking asthma.

The role of the physiotherapist

Physiotherapists are usually attached to hospitals, but some health centres employ one. They are especially good at communicating the skills needed to control asthma, such as the proper use of inhalers. They can discuss the trigger factors and teach correct breathing and relaxation. They can also show how the asthmatic can be taught to tolerate exercise.

The habit of relaxation and relaxed breathing, learnt when free of an asthmatic attack, can be a great help in the earlier stages of an attack. Relaxation can be either general or local. By general relaxation the physiotherapist means letting go of each muscle one by one, starting with the toes and working up through the whole body, so that all tension slips away. You may ask whether this cannot be achieved in sleep. But we may sleep in a way that is tense and unrelaxed, and sleep does not remove all tension. Local relaxation is aimed at the shoulders and chest muscles and teaches you to check whether these are as relaxed as you suppose.

Some years ago I went to the Brompton Hospital in London to make a film for doctors about breathing exercises. The superintendent physiotherapist told me that I would be the first to benefit: 'You are a shallow breather,' she told me. I have read recently that I probably share this characteristic with most of the population: we simply fail to use our lungs properly, breathing only with the upper part of the lungs and leaving the old stale air in the lower part. In contrast dogs, cats and other non-human animals generally take full breaths every time, to their great advantage. Diaphragmatic breathing, out of fashion in some medical circles, is welcomed by mothers as something they can teach to their asthmatic child. It consists in learning to breathe gently, not a deep breath, from the bottom of the lungs.

What scientists do not endorse is the idea that we can be usefully trained to move one part of the chest independently of all the other parts. In practice, the accessory muscles (those between the ribs and, during exercise, around the neck and shoulders) are brought into play just as and when we need them.

In severe asthma there may be an excess of secretions in the lungs; a physiotherapist can teach 'postural drainage' to help clear this and make breathing easier. A lying position on a firm support, tilted to provide the drainage, is accompanied by one or two 'huffs' to help move the secretions from the lower to the upper air passages.

Over-breathing

This should not be confused with the faster breathing that is needed in an attack to provide sufficient oxygen when deeper breathing is not possible. Over-breathing means 'hyper-ventilation', or breathing at a greater rate than the body needs at the time. In asthmatics this panting is sometimes attributed to their understandable anxiety, wrongly described sometimes as 'panic'. It may simply mean being out of breath through exercise taken when we are unfit.

When the rate of breathing is increased in this way, there is no significant increase in the take-up of oxygen by the blood, but it can reduce the waste gas, carbon dioxide, to an excessive extent. This has many undesirable results because carbon dioxide is not simply a by-product of respiration, it is also a regulator of the central nervous system. If the pressure of carbon dioxide in the blood falls to a small extent, through just a moderate degree of over-breathing, this results in a speeding up of nervous impulses, an increase in sympathetic activity (the 'fight or flight' response) which dilates the breathing tubes, and hearing and sight become more acute. If, however, the carbon dioxide pressure falls to a severe extent, these reactions are reversed. This results in a slowing of brain function and an increase in parasympathetic activity. This leads not only to dizziness, headache, cramp, sweating and a feeling of anxiety but also to a constriction of the airways. If over-breathing continues for a few minutes, the automatic impulse to breathe is switched off and the patient turns blue. Occasionally children use this ruse to frighten their parents and get their own way.

The remedy for hyper-ventilation is to practise controlled breathing in the non-asthmatic state. In a very severe attack, however, voluntary control of the breathing rate may be impossible.

One consequence of over-breathing helps to explain how in tribal ceremonies the initiates are able to endure mutilation and other trials. The dancing, singing and excitement of the ceremony leads to hyper-ventilation and after a time this can decrease the sensation of pain.

Getting excited or upset

That emotion can cause breathlessness will be accepted by anyone who has choked with laughter, become breathless with excitement or had to make a speech in public. In normal people such wheezy responses are short-lived, but in asthmatics they may be prolonged. This response may be due to the cool air acting on the nerves which lie under leaky airway linings, or to over-breathing. However, scientists have recently demonstrated that a disturbing experience can increase airway obstruction even when the rate of breathing remains normal.

We might expect the opposite result, since the sympathetic system's 'fight or flight' response prepares the body for action by opening the airways, and adrenaline is released in response to stress. However, it may be that anxiety, especially when prolonged, tends to constrict the airways. Asthmatics are certainly aware that at times the illness feeds on itself by the patient worrying about an attack which is developing, say when we have gone out for a drive and left the inhaler behind. On the way back, when relief is in prospect, the wheezing may diminish. And when we are wholly absorbed in a creative pursuit we forget about the wheezes altogether!

Much has been written about the way emotions may reinforce an attack of asthma. Little has been said about the devastating way in which asthma can spoil relations with other people. This will be one of the topics reserved for Chapter Nine on page 168.

The mysterious effect of the atmosphere

Even non-asthmatics are aware that the weather can raise or depress their spirits; but asthmatics, with their super-sensitive airways, can react to quite small changes in weather conditions. Some are particularly upset by cold damp airstreams, others by hot dry weather. Summer thunderstorms make them reach for their inhalers, and so do autumn mists. In severe asthma, changes of temperature indoors, even by a few degrees, can intensify an attack.

Scientists are not certain why changes in temperature and humidity can have such a marked effect on asthma, though they warn us not to live near rivers or over underground streams in cities. These changes are closely bound up with the behaviour of the living allergens. Pollens are released in sunny weather, moulds in damp weather; and the seasons play their part. When the hay and corn are harvested, countless millions of mould spores are released into the air and drift over country and town alike. So the explanation as to why changes in the weather can affect asthma are many and various. The following ideas will at least illustrate some of the links between the two.

• As was explained above in Chapter One, 'Why do I have asthma?', all our airways, upper and lower, are protected by a mucus blanket which is propelled upwards and outwards by tiny cilial hairs. In a dry atmosphere the blanket may disappear, exposing the sensitive tissues beneath. This is why central heating can contribute to wheeziness.

• Cold air drives people indoors, where they are exposed to house dust mites and swap infections.

• Moulds are active in warm damp weather. This is when they release their spores.

• Damp weather is associated with low clouds and these prevent polluted air from rising. If at the same time the prevailing wind is blowing the smoke from a power station towards us, this can cause our airways to react.

• We have seen that chest infections can trigger or worsen attacks of asthma. No less than ninety-five per cent of these are caused by virus colds, and these in turn are triggered by cold damp weather. The viruses live all the time in our upper breathing passages; it is the weather which causes them to multiply.

On 7 July 1983 a tremendous thunderstorm banged its way over Birmingham, England. Asthmatics were rushed into the hospitals, mostly between 9 p.m. and 6 a.m. Dr Jon Ayres has reported on the possible causes for their attacks: it might have been the falling air pressure, or a 'temperature inversion' (warm air on top of cooler air) with zero wind speed and the airborne allergens unable to rise. (There was certainly a huge release of mould spores into the thundery rain flurries.) Or it could have been a build-up in the atmosphere of oxides of nitrogen and of positive ions (discussed below under 'ionizers'), or some other factor as yet unrecorded. Or it may have been a combination of some or all of these elements which filled the emergency beds.

Ionizers and strange winds

In Southern Europe in the summer, hot dry winds come from Africa which make people edgy and bad-tempered. In Bavaria there is a notorious wind which puts up the homicide rate. Scientists state that these winds are heavily charged with positive 'ions', tiny particles which can carry a positive or negative electrical charge. They also believe that positive ions can increase the amount of a hormone in the blood called serotonin, and that this is responsible for the ill effects, including a narrowing of the airways. These arguments are used commercially to support the sale of negative ionizers. Unfortunately, up to now, no one has been able to demonstrate that they do anything to prevent the attacks, possibly because they are too local in their output, but more probably because there are so many other trigger factors in asthma in addition to negative ions. It is best to try one out before buying it.

Fog and filthy air

I well remember the 'pea-soupers', the smogs which affected our big cities before the Clean Air Act was passed in 1956 and created the smoke-free zones. The smog was a combination of dense fog and smoke, trapped close to the ground because of a sudden fall in temperature. The smoke came from the domestic coal fires, not from industry, and was responsible, during the great London smog of December 1952, for some 4,000 deaths from asthma and bronchitis.

Air pollution has been a trigger for asthma for many years; and this was recognized by Sir John Floyer in 1698 in his *Treatise on Asthma*:

> Any kind of smoak offends the spirits of the Afthmatic, and for that reafon many of them cannot bear the Air of London, whofe Smoak, like Fire it felf, irritates their Spirits into an Expanfion.

Our present-day 'clean air' may be deceptive. Our power stations still fill the air with fumes; lorries and motor cars emitting noxious gases multiply in our streets. In the countryside farmers spray crops with toxic chemicals and create clouds of smoke when they fire their straw stubble, to the great distress of the asthmatics who dwell nearby. Below are listed only a few of the many pollutants released into our atmosphere:

- sulphur dioxide

This is a powerful irritant for asthmatics and is let loose into the atmosphere whenever carbon fuels are burned, as for example in coal- or oil-fired power stations. If you have to live in a city, it is clearly advisable to be located between the prevailing source of wind (usually the south-west) and the smoke stacks.

- motor vehicle exhausts

Cars and lorries emit nitrogen oxides. The ultra-violet light in sunlight acts on these to produce ozone. Contrary to popular belief, ozone is highly irritant.

- smoke and fumes from fires

The smoke from a domestic wood fire (or bonfire) and the fumes from a leaky stove can provoke asthma. Central heating (with added humidity) is preferable, augmented by local electric heaters.

NO SMOKING please!

So far as many asthmatics are concerned, cigar and cigarette smoke can be the worst form of air pollution. The airways of asthma sufferers are exquisitely sensitive to the smoke exhaled by others. Nevertheless many asthmatics find they cannot bring themselves to give up the habit: almost as many are smokers (about twenty-five per cent) as in the population at large (thirty per cent all told).

Why is cigarette smoke bad for asthmatics, whether inhaled actively or passively? Many people with asthma continue to smoke either to calm their nerves or because the smoke helps them cough up their phlegm. This latter function happens because the mucus glands respond to the smoke by increasing their output. At the same time, however, the smoke irritates those sensitive nerves lying just beneath the linings of the airways (leaky linings when we are asthmatic), and this sends a signal to the bronchial muscles to thicken so that the airways narrow. At the same time it paralyses the cilia which, as we have seen, are designed to waft the mucus blanket up and away out of the lungs. The extra mucus stays in the airways, waiting for the invading germs which thrive and multiply and set up their own chain reaction, and this ends up in more signals to those twitchy airway muscles.

That is the asthmatic's response to cigarette smoke. In time the procedure may damage the walls of the airways and spread into the air sacs (alveoli) where the gases are exchanged. The lungs become less and less capable of defending themselves against invading bacteria (including some that are normally quite harmless). Antibiotics may be used, but these become decreasingly effective. This is the condition known as chronic bronchitis, which is not reversible and fills hospital beds with people on an inexorable and wretched downhill slide.

This leads to the inevitable conclusion that smoking should be cut out altogether. How this can be done is beyond the scope of this book, but useful advice can be obtained from the Health Education Authority and from A.S.H., whose addresses are given under 'Useful Addresses'. There are four stages in the process of giving up smoking:

1 Think of all the reasons for stopping

2 Decide how smoking is linked to certain habits

3 Choose a BIG DAY and cut out smoking altogether

4 Do not slip back, and reward success by giving your family a treat with the money you have saved.

If you are an employer who wants to impose a ban on smoking there are three rules you must bear in mind: consult the workforce; announce and publicize the policy in advance; make emergency arrangements for smokers who cannot give up immediately.

There is an alternative to smoking. About a million people in Britain now take snuff. This habit does no damage to the lungs or to the nasal passages and apparently provides uplift. Chewing gum containing nicotine is another alternative to smoking.

Home sweet home

Having done our best to frustrate dust, animal dander, smokers and mould spores, we are still left with some nagging worries about the air we breathe inside our homes. What is the ideal temperature? And the ideal humidity?

What helps those asthmatics who are especially sensitive to changes in air temperature (even to a fall of a few degrees) is a fairly even temperature all day throughout the home, but which is of course allowed to fall at night. In these days of efficient central heating this is not hard to achieve, even in countries such as Finland where in winter the outside temperature drops to well below freezing. Unfortunately it is hard to manage this without providing an ideal climate for the house dust mite and making the atmosphere too dry, so drying up the mucus blanket which protects the breathing passages, leaving them exposed to irritants and the cold air when we step outside. This can be overcome with the help of humidifiers attached to the central heating radiators, or a dish of water kept near the gas or electric fire. It is also possible to buy a humidifying machine, but this has to be cleaned frequently to prevent asthma-provoking moulds from forming in the ducts. A dehumidifier is used by some people to frustrate the growth of moulds which flourish in damp air.

One of the reasons why we get more colds in winter is that we congregate together in airless rooms and exchange germs. On the other hand, the cold virus multiplies less by direct contact than as a result of falls in the temperature which lower our resistance to it. The conclusion to be drawn from all this is that we have to work out what inside conditions suit us best by trial and error and then try to persuade everyone else to adapt to them – not an easy task since people have very firm views about the kind of atmosphere that suits them, be they healthy or asthmatic. The scientists will need to leave their laboratories and start to investigate our homes before we can gain any really convincing picture as to what makes an ideal home for a wheezy person.

Some drugs can cause asthma

It is not generally realized that some drugs can cause severe asthma. One group of these is connected with aspirin, and sensitivity to aspirin is especially associated with those asthmatics who also develop nasal polyps. Many drugs which can be bought over the counter for colds, headaches and rheumatism contain aspirin; an asthmatic who is sensitive to aspirin should consult the retail pharmacist before making a purchase. NSAIDs (non-steroidal anti-inflammatory drugs), for example 'Ibuprofen' and 'Indomethacin' (which is used for severe back pain), can also cause severe asthma in aspirin-sensitive people.

Among the many drugs used to treat high blood pressure, there is a group called the 'beta-blocker' drugs. These can initiate asthma in people sensitive to them, and the resultant illness can be so severe as to cause death. Eye-drops containing a beta-blocker, sometimes used in cases of glaucoma, should also be avoided since there have been cases of death being caused by asthma following the placing of one drop in each eye.

Chemicals and additives

Many asthmatics find that their asthma gets worse when the walls of their homes have just been painted and are giving off solvent fumes. Other chemicals used in the home which can make asthmatics wheeze include air fresheners, hair sprays, fly sprays, talcum powder and washing powder which contains enzymes. Solvents are not only used to thin paints, in the form of white spirit, but are also used in dry cleaning and carpet-cleaning fluids and in many glues. Dieldrin moth proofer is released by solvents, and wood preservatives based on Lindane or PLP produce a vapour which can cause wheeziness. (It is alarming to read that some solvents can react with the flames from a gas fire to produce phosgene gas!)

It can happen that a person with only mild or latent asthma can be overwhelmed by exposure to a chemical additive, and from then on become 'hyper-responsive' to triggers present in quite small quantities. Some chemicals are hidden but can still cause trouble, for example the formaldehyde in chipboard used by the office furniture industry. Some local authorities provide an environmental health service, which includes a Home Check Scheme designed to point out possible health hazards.

A particularly distressing form of asthma is that which arises directly from a person's occupation, for example in the bakery trade or as a hairdresser. This is discussed in Chapter Six, 'Asthma related to work'. Mothers of asthmatic children have their own special concern: they worry about the many chemical additives which are now included in our manufactured foods, a topic which is treated in Chapter Seven.

Infections

It is a common experience among asthmatics that coughs and colds make their asthma worse – indeed, may provoke an attack in the first place. Some people have asthma only when they have a cold, or at least they believe this to be the case. Some virus attacks produce no asthma.

The cold is typically caused by a rhinovirus ('rhino' being medical jargon for the nose). These viruses can easily descend to the breathing tubes and act as irritants, or may contribute to the breakdown of the linings of the breathing tubes if there is a severe infection. The presence of viruses can make the airways more 'twitchy', more responsive to other irritants.

Bacteria may arrive as well; and these can stimulate the production of antibodies, as well as producing histamine themselves. There may be present, especially in older people, a bronchitis which causes the production of phlegm and it is often difficult for either doctor or patient to decide whether it is the asthma or the bronchitis which is the major cause of phlegm.

Infection is particularly likely to precipitate asthma in infants and young children with the synctial virus predominating, and in older adults. Feverish, influenza-like illnesses which do not have the symptoms of a head cold are generally less provoking. Other infections such as measles, chicken-pox and diarrhoea do not trigger attacks of asthma.

It is important for the distinction between 'asthma' and various forms of bronchitis to be made clear to the patient. A diagnosis of 'bronchitis' by itself is not a diagnosis at all, since the term simply means an 'itis' (inflammation) of the bronchi (breathing tubes) and so includes both asthma (when there is inflammation) and acute and chronic bronchitis. 'Wheezy bronchitis' is just another name for asthma, designed to hide the true nature of the illness.

The differences between these similar illnesses can be summarized in a table:

| | BRONCHITIS | | |
	acute	chronic	wheezy = ASTHMA
wheeziness		*	**
inflammation	**	**	**
infection	**	**	*
caused by smoking		**	−
treated with antibiotics	**		
treated with anti-asthma drugs		*	**
** = usually * = sometimes − = not initially			

Doctors sometimes prescribe an antibiotic when there is an infection. This is not aimed at the virus, against which it is powerless, nor will it directly lessen the asthmatic response. It is aimed at the secondary infection which can, as we have seen, trigger this response. This argument is taken further in Chapter Three, 'Other medicines', on page 82.

Some parents take the idealistic view that they should try to shield their children completely from exposure to infections. This is clearly impossible, especially when the child starts going to school. On the contrary, school games and exercises are essential in the achievement of physical fitness, and this, together with warm clothes and a balanced diet, will help build resistance to the viruses. If the head colds are very numerous, then allergic rhinitis may be suspected and should be treated as such.

As an older asthmatic, I take the precaution of avoiding going into crowded places such as theatres and cinemas in the months when they are likely to attract people full of coughs and sneezes, since I find I pick up infection very easily, and changes in temperature, from cold street to warm theatre, can encourage the cold viruses. In adults, asthma can be provoked by Influenza 'A' virus, so if you have severe chronic asthma it is a good plan to ask your doctor to inoculate you against influenza early in October or November when the vaccine becomes available.

Asthma at night

It is commonly believed that most asthmatics find their cough or wheeze is worst at night, or when waking, usually after 3 a.m. This is often referred to as 'the early morning dip', that is to say, a dip in the reading of peak flow (before any correcting medicine is taken).

Virtually all asthmatics, of all ages, have episodes of early morning tightness; a recent survey of 7,000 asthmatics revealed that about two-thirds experience it as often as three times a week. This has led doctors to use night wheeziness or cough as a sign that the patient may indeed have asthma – though bronchitics may also remove phlegm in this way. Since loss of sleep can affect performance during the following day, and since night asthma is the major cause of hospital referrals in asthma, it is essential that it should be controlled and prevented if at all possible.

Why do asthmatics wheeze at night? Various theories have been put forward:

· In the seventeenth century Sir Thomas Willis ascribed it to 'an overheating of the blood by the bed clothes'. Nowadays physicians know that the blood temperature remains constant, but they are aware that the house dust mite likes to live in bed linen (especially in wool and feathers), and to feed on the tiny skin scales which humans shed at night. But many asthmatics who are not allergic to house dust mite nevertheless have night asthma, so there must be some other explanation.

· Another factor could be the 'late allergic reaction' described in the last chapter. But not all asthmatics are allergic and second phase attacks are not nearly as common as night asthma.

· It is tempting to suppose that night asthma is simply due to the fact that the aerosol bronchodilator taken at 11 p.m. has no effect after 3 a.m. But some patients wheeze in the early hours even when a bronchodilator is used frequently at intervals during the night.

· At night, the clearance of mucus through the beating of the cilia greatly decreases during sleep, so there is likely to be a build-up of allergens and irritants in the mucus. This may contribute, but it is not believed to be the major factor. Scientists also view the cooling of the airways at night to be too slight to be significant, especially when the room temperature is well maintained.

· Until recently it was thought that the changes in the supply of hormones which take place at night (they drop just as the peak flow drops), especially corticosteroids, could explain night asthma. However, these hormones are made by the adrenal glands, and in asthmatics the drop in peak flow still takes place even when the glands have been removed (for other reasons).

There remains one possible explanation: that sleep is the cause of night asthma. In 1698 Sir John Floyer seems to have had the same opinion: 'I have observed,' he wrote, 'that Fits of Asthma seem always to happen after Sleep in the Night, when the nerves are filled with windy Spirits.' It has been shown in shift workers that the time their airways narrow is when they are asleep, and this has been reproduced in studies in which asthmatics are kept awake one night and allowed to sleep the next.

It is not a 'windy spirit' which is responsible but the circadian rhythms. In every human being, sleep brings with it a slight reduction in the heart rate, in blood pressure and in the diameter of the airways. In asthmatics these narrow to a much greater extent, and their peak flow starts from a lower level anyway. Their airways do not become more twitchy at night but are sufficiently twitchy at all times to produce this effect, to the point where cough and wheeze is experienced. The circadian rhythms are partly mediated by the vagus nerve, and if this is blocked by the use of ipratropium (Atrovent) then the airways constrict to a lesser extent.

It is therefore sensible to treat night asthma by reducing twitchiness at all times with the use of preventive medicine. And if this is not sufficient, then a slow-release bronchodilator can be effective. One of these is theophylline but it tends to diminish sleep; the hunt is on for a slow-release bronchodilator which does not have this effect, 'salmeterol' being a promising candidate which is under trial.

Chapter Three

MANAGING ASTHMA WITH MEDICINES

The principles of treatment

The aim of treatment should be that the asthmatic remains free from symptoms at all times and leads a normal life. This implies an ability both to abort the sudden acute attack and to damp down the inflammation. The fact that at present this is not always achieved suggests that the pharmaceutical companies have a long road to travel before they will be able to claim that they can provide totally effective remedies. (That they are working hard on our behalf is evidenced by the fact that since I began writing this book in May 1987 three new ways of taking our medicines have been introduced.) Sooner or later the *perfect* anti-inflammatory agent will be developed and no other medicine will be needed.

What the present medicines do quite well is to block the action of triggers of all kinds so that the following reactions are avoided or reversed:

- a thickening of the airway muscles
- a swelling of the linings of the airways

No single medicine will deal with all the asthmatic reactions. It is convenient to divide anti-asthma medicines into three groups: 'relievers', 'preventers' and 'acute savers' and they will be described under these headings later in this chapter. The first two groups may be summarized as follows:

RELIEVERS	PREVENTERS
THE SWORD:	THE SHIELD:
AIM: to relieve constriction by relaxing the airway muscles	AIM: to prevent or reverse the inflammation
BRONCHODILATORS	ANTI-INFLAMMATORY AGENTS
(1) adrenaline derivatives	(1) steroids
e.g. salbutamol	e.g. beclomethasone
(2) caffeine derivatives	prednisolone
e.g. theophylline	hydrocortisone
(3) atropine derivatives	(2) non-steroidal
e.g. ipratroprium	e.g. nedocromil
	ketotifen
	ANTI-ALLERGIC AGENT
	e.g. sodium cromoglycate

How does the doctor choose the treatments?

Generally speaking, the 'bronchodilators' are used to relieve **acute** attacks: those which are sudden in their onset and can be quickly reversed. In persistent **chronic** asthma, the aim is to prevent attacks by using both a bronchodilator and a preventive medicine, on a regular day-to-day basis but in very small doses. This does not mean that there is permanent lung damage but that the breathing tubes have become 'hyper-responsive' to the invading triggers and need to be made less angry.

In a **severe** attack, one which does not respond to a bronchodilator at a normal dosage, the doctor will most likely give both a high dose of bronchodilator and a high dose of preventive medicine, leaving the patient to continue with the latter for a short period and then revert to whatever regular medication is seen to be appropriate.

Having diagnosed that you are suffering from asthma, the doctor adopts the following principles. He at first prescribes the lowest dose and the shortest course of treatment, using the safest route, that matches all the data he has gathered about your attacks. (Four case-histories are given in Chapter Four, 'How does the doctor choose the treatments?', to illustrate the way the medicines have to be adjusted to the severity and frequency of the attacks.) You may return after a few days or weeks and report that the treatment has been ineffective. This may be due to one or more of a number of reasons:

• The medicine was not taken correctly.

• It was used properly, but you could not accept the side effects and gave up.

• The dosage was too low (either too small a dose or one that was taken too infrequently).

• The form in which the drug was taken was not suitable. (Medicines can be taken in many ways: they can be swallowed as syrups or tablets; inhaled as a powder or as droplets from a breath-operated inhaler; or taken as a suppository by the rectal route.)

• The medicine managed to relieve symptoms during the day but was not effective at night because it was short-acting.

• It worked well in relieving spasm but needed additionally to be assisted by an anti-inflammatory agent.

The doctor recognizes that no two patients are alike in the way they respond to a particular treatment. This is because people vary in their ability to absorb the drugs and, hence, in the degree to which the drugs will cause side effects. They also vary in the extent to which they are able to understand and comply with the instructions that have been given.

It follows that doctors have to proceed by trial and error; they depend very much on the patient's description of the symptoms. These may have disappeared by the time the consultation takes place, typically in the late afternoon when asthma is usually at its mildest. The doctor may therefore ask the patient to take a series of measurements of 'peak expiratory air flow' by blowing hard into a **peak flow meter** in the way described in Chapter Four, 'The invaluable peak flow meter'. This will help the doctor to decide the severity and nature of the attacks and to adjust treatment accordingly.

Do the medicines become less effective with repeated use?

Most of the drugs used nowadays have been tested over twenty years, and there is little evidence that they become less effective when used day after day and month after month. There is one possible exception: the adrenaline derivatives may become less effective after two weeks of continuous use if there is chronic asthma and inhaled steroids are not used at the same time.

If the medicines seem to be becoming less effective than before, this is because the asthma has deteriorated (so that a higher dose is needed, or a different bronchodilator or additional steroids). It is unwise for the patient to keep increasing the dose if it seems not to be working, and the doctor should be consulted at an early opportunity.

How safe are the treatments?

Nearly all medicines have 'side effects': they cause reactions in the body which by themselves do not bring the required benefit. We must not confuse side effects which are dangerously toxic with those that are merely unpleasant. Some of the medicines used to treat asthma can cause reactions which are upsetting, for example a nervous tremor. Even when severe, these reactions are not necessarily dangerous, but they may result in the patient asking for an alternative treatment. Patients vary a good deal in their reactions to medicines and doctors have to take this into account when prescribing.

As far as safety is concerned, we should distinguish between the remedies available up to the 1970s and those which have been introduced since. Before the 1970s we had theophylline, which is toxic at about twice the treatment dose; isoprenaline, which can upset heart rhythms; and we had tablet steroids which, if taken in high doses over long periods, can have debilitating effects.

Since that time, new ways of taking the older drugs have been introduced and new medicines, which are either exceptionally safe or can be given in doses which avoid the toxic effects. These developments will be explained in detail in the following pages.

At this stage, we can note the ways in which the scientists have improved the element of safety:

• They have re-formulated drugs so that only the active ingredient is included while the harmful ingredients are excluded (for example, the bronchodilators such as salbutamol, which can admittedly give people 'the shakes' but which, though unpleasant, are not in themselves dangerous).

• They have devised inhalers of various kinds which deliver the drug directly to the air passages so that it does not need to travel round the body first before reaching its destination. As a result, only tiny doses are needed. These inhalers are available for most types of drugs used in asthma, the exceptions being the theophyllines and ketotifen.

• They have devised increasingly ingenious slow-release forms of drugs taken as tablets, so that a small dose is delivered continuously rather than a big one all at once. This has rescued the theophyllines and also been applied with sophistication to salbutamol.

• They have managed to introduce radically new drugs (such as sodium cromoglycate and nedocromil) which have no significant side effects.

None of the medicines properly used in the treatment of asthma is a drug of addiction in the sense in which it is possible to become addicted to morphine or to certain tranquillizers. There have been cases in which teenagers have become addicted to the freon propellant used in a metered-dose aerosol inhaler – the remedy for which is to switch to an inhaler which delivers in the form of a powder, as described below, in 'A closer look at inhalers'.

Another question that is often raised is: 'Can I take more than one medicine at a time, or will this increase the side effects?' The opposite may be the case, because it is often possible to reduce the dose of one type of drug if another is used as well, assuming that the second operates through a different route within the airways. This will be explained in the pages which follow.

How are the drugs given?

This will be discussed in more detail in 'A closer look at inhalers' on page 83. For our present purposes, the methods available can be divided quite simply into two general types:

	TAKEN AT HOME	GIVEN BY THE DOCTOR
The drug circulates in the bloodstream	tablets capsules syrups	injections
The drug is directed into the air passages	aerosols powders spacer nebulizer	nebulizer

Each method has its advantages and disadvantages. If the drug has to circulate round the bloodstream before it reaches the air passages, it will enter all parts of the body and produce responses where they are not needed. On the other hand, if the air passages are blocked, this may be the most effective route. Tablets can be modified to provide slow release over an extended period, and this can help relieve night-time attacks.

It is generally more effective to deliver the drug directly to the air passages by inhaling it, and any side effects are likely to be greatly reduced thereby. To increase the effectiveness, a device such as a spacer can be fitted to the inhaler. To deal with a severe attack, the doctor can inject a large dose via the bloodstream or use a nebulizer, which enables a continuous stream of fine particles of the drug to be inhaled.

When choosing between these methods, the doctor has to take into account the age of the patient, the type of asthma, the probable triggers and the seriousness of the attacks. The patient's own preferences also have to be considered. At first the wide choice of routes and devices can seem bewildering, but there is one great advantage: if one method fails to give relief then another can be tried, so the patient should never give up but insist that an effective method be found.

Some of the drugs (for example, salbutamol) are available in all forms. Theophylline is restricted to tablets, injections and suppositories. Steroids can be taken in many different ways, but sodium cromoglycate can be taken only by the inhaled route. The forms in which the different drugs are available are listed in Appendix E, on page 208.

What is meant by the 'placebo' effect?

Some asthmatics react favourably to treatments which have no proven therapeutic value. Such treatments are said to have a 'placebo' effect as, for example, when inert substances are given in clinical trials as a means of comparing the response when active drugs are used. This suggests that there are asthmatics, clearly a minority, in whom the power of suggestion is strong, and this is one of the reasons why doctors may be reluctant to change a course of treatment which has become out-dated, if the patient feels benefit from it. The converse is also true, that if for any reason a patient resents the treatment that has been prescribed, it is unlikely to be fully effective, even though backed by the evidence of numerous clinical trials.

Relievers, Preventers and Acute Savers

Group A: 'Relievers'

The aim: to relax the smooth muscles which control the diameter of the air passages (bronchi) and so relieve the spasm. Recent research has confirmed that bronchodilators have no effect on the inflammation of the airways.

There is a wide choice of bronchodilators, each available in many forms. They divide into three groups:

A1 adrenaline derivatives
salbutamol ('Ventolin', 'Volmax', 'Aerolin')
terbutaline ('Bricanyl')
fenoterol ('Berotec')

A2 caffeine derivatives
aminophylline ('Phyllocontin')
theophylline ('Nuelin', 'Theodur')

A3 atropine derivative
ipratropium ('Atrovent')

A1 *adrenaline derivatives*

Before the Second World War, adrenaline (given by injection) and ephedrine (taken as a tablet) were the only drugs available for relieving an asthma attack. They did so by reversing spasm of the muscles surrounding the airways, and did their job very efficiently. Unfortunately, they had undesirable effects as well: a racing pulse, anxiety and excitement. The scientists in the pharmaceutical companies spent a lot of time after the war looking for derivatives of adrenaline which would relieve the spasm without stimulating the heart muscles. Their first achievement was to bring out an aerosol inhaler with metered doses; these could be very small because they reached the air passages directly and did not need to travel round the body. Unfortunately, the drug used, isoprenaline, also stimulated the nervous system.

The big breakthrough came soon afterwards when airway-dilating drugs were developed; these latched on to the Beta 2 receptors in the airway muscles but had no effect on the heart muscles. They are often referred to as 'beta-agonists' or agents which are 'sympathomimetic' because they stimulate at least part of the response of the sympathetic nervous system, which dilates the airways. The approved names are those shown in the above table: salbutamol, terbutaline and fenoterol.

It must be emphasized that this group of drugs only relieves muscle spasm in the airways; there is no reduction of inflammation or any effect on 'twitchiness' (the way the airways respond to irritants). So they are used mainly as 'relievers' rather than as 'preventers'. However, when taken before exercise or on a regular four-hourly basis, they can at least be said to be preventing the muscle spasm.

How are they taken?

There are various ways in which these adrenaline derivatives can be taken at home. They can be swallowed as syrups, or as tablets which can incorporate a slow-release facility. They can be inhaled as dry powders or with aerosol sprays; the sprays can be provided with tube spacers or large volume spacers. They can be inhaled from nebulizers which are driven by compressed air. These forms are available for other medicines used in asthma; their function will be described later in this chapter. The doctor has an additional route for administration: he can inject directly into the bloodstream, under the skin or into a muscle. But it is now more common for a doctor to use a nebulizer to give a high dose in an acute attack.

As far as the adrenaline derivatives are concerned, the inhaled forms possess advantages over the syrups and tablets. When taken from a metered-dose inhaler (either as an aerosol spray or as a dry powder) there is fast relief, usually within five minutes. The dose is very small and can be repeated whenever needed to relieve wheeziness. The pocket inhaler is convenient: it can be carried around anywhere and used before exercise or exposure to cold air.

The pocket inhalers do have some disadvantages. Young children find them difficult to use and so are often given a syrup instead. The inhaler does not work very well if the airways are blocked with debris, though this situation arises only when the attack is really severe. The aerosol inhaler has the additional problem for the very young and for the elderly that it requires good co-ordination between squeezing and breathing, and some youngsters can become addicted to the freon propellant.

These disadvantages can be overcome if a dry powder inhaler is used. This delivers the same particle sizes into the airways, at a slightly higher dosage; the powder is sucked in. The same principle is used in the newly introduced disc-inhaler, which provides salbutamol in numbered doses. Another device which has been launched to overcome the problem of co-ordination when an aerosol is used is the 'auto-inhaler' which also delivers salbutamol when the patient breathes in.

The adrenaline derivatives can also be taken as tablets. These avoid the problem of co-ordination and the resistance offered by blocked airways. On the other hand, tablets are more likely to give rise to what patients describe as 'the shakes' – a tremor of the hands, excitability in children and a racing pulse. These unwanted effects are diminished if the tablets incorporate a slow-release principle which extends the active life of the dose to about eight hours (compared with only four hours when a pocket inhaler is used). Traditional forms include Ventolin Spandets and Bricanyl S A, with a newer slow-release preparation now available for salbutamol called Volmax. The aim of Volmax is to release the drug at a constant rate over twelve hours so that only two tablets need be taken every twenty-four hours to provide a continuous dosage.

The slow-release tablets provide salbutamol or similar drug at a level about 40–80 times that of the dose from a metered inhaler. Therefore it may well happen that, although tremor is experienced with the tablet forms, it is avoided with the inhalers, always assuming they are used correctly. A table of the doses provided by the different devices is given in Appendix D.

Some controversy surrounds the use of nebulizers. These deliver a large dose in the form of a mist which can be inhaled even when the patient is breathing only with difficulty. Doctors use them to relieve a severe attack. They are sometimes given to parents to administer when their children have severe and persistent asthma, or to adults for a limited period. Their great disadvantage is their very efficiency: when a nebulized bronchodilator is given, the spasm of the smooth muscle surrounding the airways is usually relieved very efficiently; but any underlying inflammation remains untreated and the airways are consequently at the risk of further attack.

Adrenaline derivatives: a summary

This group of bronchodilators is used as the first line of defence against asthma. For many asthmatics it forms the only kind of treatment that is given. The usual way of taking them is via a pocket inhaler which is carried around at all times, with reserve inhalers placed in strategic locations, such as in the glove pocket of the car, under the pillow and in a drawer at the office.

These bronchodilators act fast to relieve airway constriction of the smooth muscles, whether touched off by exercise or by an allergic reaction. They are either used as needed to reverse an attack, or on a regular basis (three or four times a day) to provide a continuous dose, or through a slow-release tablet which is especially useful at night-time. They have no effect on inflammation or excessive secretion in the airways.

The inhaled bronchodilators tend to be under-used, probably because of the warnings on the packets and the containers: 'it is dangerous to exceed the stated dose'. This warning is surprising in view of the very small dose that is delivered and the fact that no one has ever died as a result of an overdose of these drugs, taken in any form. The 'shakes' are alarming but not dangerous; and it may be possible to bring a moderately severe attack under control by increasing the inhaled dose.

The reason for the restriction is partly to protect the manufacturers, but mainly because the need to take more and more inhalations really means that you should be consulting the doctor, because the asthma is not being properly controlled. He may well prescribe in addition a treatment to deal with the inflammation, and possibly a slow-release form to help cope with the night asthma.

There are three important rules to observe:

• Learn how to use the inhaler correctly, so that you get enough medicine into your lungs.

• Use the inhaler as soon as you feel an attack coming on.

• Take the doses that have been recommended by your doctor; if they do not bring relief, obtain fresh medical advice. (See especially the section in Chapter Four on 'What you should do if things go wrong', page 110.)

A2 *caffeine derivatives:* ✒ *The theophyllines (xanthines)*

Theophylline occurs naturally in tea and coffee and is closely related to caffeine. It has been said that the stimulant action of caffeine was first discovered by an Arabian monk, who noticed that goats which had eaten berries from coffee plants became extra frisky. Caffeine has been used to treat wheeziness for hundreds of years, but only in this century has the active substance, theophylline, been identified. Aminophylline is a soluble form of the same drug, and is the one that used to be used for injection, a way of dealing with a severe attack, but which has given way to salbutamol and terbutaline given from a nebulizer.

Theophylline, like the adrenaline derivatives, is used to give relief from bronchospasm and has no effect on inflammation. The two groups of drugs act by different routes (no one knows exactly how they act), and they are sometimes used in combination to provide a stronger action.

Theophylline has two main disadvantages. It cannot be taken from an inhaler because this causes coughing, which makes the asthma worse. The second problem is that it is not selective and affects all the tissues in the body, not only the breathing tubes but also the heart, brains, kidneys and the stomach. Some patients cannot tolerate it at all, even in very small doses, while others find that they can obtain relief at a dosage which does not produce the nausea, the stomach pains, the headache, the sleepless nights and the emotional disturbance.

In spite of these disadvantages, theophylline is widely used in countries where the adrenaline derivatives have only recently become widely available. It had a new lease of life when the drug companies were able to bring out slow-release forms. One way in which this is achieved is to store the drug particles in a miniature wax honeycomb which is encased in a plastic coating that is gradually removed by bile acid so that the drug is slowly absorbed from the intestine. Brand names of slow-release theophylline include Nuelin S A, Slo-Phyllin, Phyllocontin Continus and Sabidal S R.

The two advantages of slow-release theophylline tablets are: they can provide twenty-four-hour cover with only two doses, and they can be used to control the symptoms of night asthma. The adrenaline derivatives (salbutamol, etc.), often additionally with inhaled steroids, are tried first; if symptoms persist, then slow-release theophylline is used, if well tolerated. Since the amount released at any given moment is small, side effects are reduced (compared with those produced by the old crystalline forms). On the Continent the drug is often given as a suppository. This reduces stomach irritation but can cause bowel irritation instead, and the dose which is effectively absorbed is unpredictable.

There is one important way in which theophylline differs from the adrenaline derivatives. It is less effective than they are in reversing the first phase of an allergic reaction but is much more likely to succeed in blocking the more dangerous second-phase attack. It is therefore a useful standby for anyone who does not have a 'crisis' course of steroid tablets or nebulized salbutamol at hand to deal with a moderately severe attack. In such cases it is essential to tell the doctor that theophylline had been taken, to avoid a dangerous double dosing. Any asthmatic on theophylline should take no higher dose than has been prescribed and should avoid all over-the-counter preparations, such as Do-Do or Franolyn, which also contain theophylline. The retail pharmacist will be able to advise what these are.

A3 *atropine derivatives*

My first introduction to atropine was in the form of a bottle of belladonna, prescribed by a herbalist. It tasted bitter and appeared to have no effect on my childhood asthma. Belladonna is extracted from the plant *Atropa belladonna*, more commonly known as deadly nightshade. Fashionable ladies used to take a tincture as eye-drops to dilate their pupils, hence the name of the plant. A modern derivative of atropine, ipratropium, is prescribed today. It is used only from an inhaler or nebulizer, and it has a bitter taste. There are two brand names: Atrovent and Duovent. Duovent is a combination of ipratropium and salbutamol.

The effect of taking the drug is to relax the bronchial muscles when they are in the thickened state and constricting the airways; and it does this by blocking the vagus nerve. This is the nerve that carries 'parasympathetic' impulses to the lungs and makes the airway muscles contract. By blocking acetylcholine (the vagus nerve transmitter), it manages to block the reflex which tightens the airway muscles. This is why this group of drugs is referred to as 'anti-cholinergic'.

As a bronchodilator, ipratropium is no better than the adrenaline derivatives already described (salbutamol, etc.). Why then is it used?

• In infants it is much more effective than the other bronchodilators.

• When used in conjunction with salbutamol, it produces a greater effect than either drug used alone, at a low dose level. Two puffs of Atrovent are taken after two puffs of Ventolin, Bricanyl or Berotec.

• It is useful in chronic bronchitis caused by smoking or infection, which suggests that the vagus nerve reflexes are important in this condition.

Group B: 'Preventers' ✳

B1 *steroids*

These are powerful drugs. It is no exaggeration to say that they have transformed the treatment of asthma when it is at least partly due to inflammation of the airways. They are used mainly as 'preventers'. They not only help to block the release of mediators from the mast cells but are believed to act at an earlier phase by preventing lymphocytes from becoming active, and in so doing block signals to the neutrophils and eosinophils which would otherwise invade the airway tissues from the bloodstream and cause the second phase of an asthmatic attack. They work at many levels to prevent asthma.

It is increasingly recognized, and is being reported at the meetings of chest physicians, that the relieving drugs which we have just considered relieve the breathlessness without controlling the asthma in general. As a result, the patient feels better; but he or she is still at risk of having another acute attack; the underlying 'twitchiness' is not relieved by the bronchodilators. To suppress asthma closer to its origins (see page 25), inhaled steroids are needed as well, if the asthma is at all persistent.

Steroids are most commonly used from inhalers. In this form they are taken every day, usually twice a day, not to reverse an attack but to reduce the likelihood of an attack taking place.

The build-up in this preventive role is slow; it may take a week or a fortnight, and this must be allowed for when the treatment is begun. It also follows that the daily dosage should be maintained even when there are no symptoms; after all, a lack of symptoms is what the treatment aims to achieve.

Steroids can also be taken as tablets by what is rather confusingly known as the 'oral route', which means that the drug enters the general circulation before it reaches the airways. This route is used in any of the following circumstances:

- to restore control when the asthma worsens

- to maintain control when the asthma is severe and persistent and all other methods have failed

- to anticipate a more than usually severe challenge to the airways, such as the onset of a bad head cold or exposure to severe weather or to allergens not usually encountered. An alternative is to increase the dosage of the inhaled form for the duration of the challenge

Steroids are also given by injection when the doctor is faced with a severe attack; and this is usually followed by a course of tablets, which ends with a decreasing dosage and is then replaced with inhaled steroid to provide daily maintenance.

Attitudes towards steroids are changing, among doctors as well as among patients. For reasons given below, it is now realized that the inhaled route is safe at the recommended doses, even when the treatment is continuous, year in and year out. The view is also gaining ground that the oral (tablet) route is safe even at a high dosage if the course of treatment is short. This has led an increasing number of physicians to give patients whose asthma is at least moderately severe a supply of tablets to start taking if they feel an attack coming on and so prevent it from becoming really bad. If they were to wait until they see their own doctor, it might be too late to stop the attack.

As recommended in Chapter Four, some asthmatics take measurements of their lung function when they feel threatened in this way; when they find that the readings on the meter are getting low, they put themselves on a short course of tablet steroids.

The steroid family

The family of steroids consists of closely related drugs which include the following commonly prescribed forms:

	Approved name	Brand names include	Dose in μ g. per puff
(Injections)	(hydrocortisone)		
Tablets	prednisone	Decortysil	
	prednisolone	Bectastab	
		Prednesol (soluble)	
Aerosol inhalers	beclomethasone dipropionate	Becotide and Becloforte	50 or 100 500
	betamethasone valerate	Bextasol	
	budesonide	Pulmicort	50 or 200
Dry powder inhalers	beclomethasone dipropionate	Becotide rotacaps and Becodisks	200

Prednisone breaks down in the body into prednisolone, and they are indistinguishable for all practical purposes. Becloforte is the same medicine as Becotide but delivers a dose which is five times stronger. This higher dosage is sometimes needed when the asthma is both severe and persistent. Becotide is itself available in two strengths, the lower one being used for children.

The advantages and disadvantages of the different kinds of inhalers will be summarized later in this chapter. By the time this book is published, it is likely that Pulmicort will also be available in a dry powder inhaler.

How safe are the steroids?

Injections of corticosteroids can save lives and are harmless. A short course of steroid tablets (e.g. prednisolone) in a high dose lasting for a week or two will not give rise to side effects, except possibly a small gain in weight, or indigestion; both effects reverse when the course has ended.

Inhaled steroids are also safe, even when taken in an extra strong form on a regular basis. This is for two reasons: because the drug is delivered directly to where it is needed, the air passages, the amount needed is very small; and in this form it has been cleverly formulated so that any part that is swallowed is broken down into harmless constituents before they enter the general circulation. Some people find that inhaled steroids irritate the throat unless they take a glass of water afterwards. A few experience a throat infection known as 'thrush', but this can be treated with lozenges. When the inhaled steroids were introduced it was found that many patients who had been taking tablet steroids for a long time could greatly reduce the dose or stop them altogether, relying entirely on the inhaled forms.

Why then has there been all the fuss about steroids? This has arisen because in illnesses such as rheumatoid arthritis, and in a decreasing number of cases of severe chronic asthma, steroids have been given as tablets in a high dose on a continuous basis. The possible side effects from this include a gain in weight, especially in the face and body. There can more rarely be a thinning of the bones and the skin. There is a heightened risk of diabetes in those prone to it.

There is another risk which occurs when prednisone is given at a level which exceeds 5 milligrams (mg) daily for more than a month or so. This makes the body's steroid-producing glands, the adrenals, lazy, so that they are not able to respond when more steroids are needed to cope with the stress of an emergency, for example an operation or illness, or an accident. Asthmatics on continuous steroids should carry a card or bracelet obtainable from Medic-Alert, to warn doctors to give extra steroids in an emergency.

Combining the treatments

Steroids do not dilate the breathing tubes but deal with the inflammation that underlies all but the very mild forms of asthma. So patients are usually advised to take an inhaled bronchodilator as well as the inhaled steroid. A typical regime is to take two puffs of inhaled bronchodilator to open the airways, followed by two puffs of inhaled steroid. This takes place before retiring and again before breakfast. Chronic asthmatics are often given inhaled steroids which, per puff, provide higher doses. At the standard dose of two puffs twice a day, these reach 1,000 micrograms (μg) (Becloforte) or 800 μg (Pulmicort), well below the 2,000 μg a day which could begin to affect the rest of the body.

If a patient has or is threatened by a severe attack which requires a course of steroid tablets in a high dose, it is usually a good plan to change gradually to the inhaled steroids in the third and fourth weeks, with the tablet dose halved and taken only on alternate days, until at the end of the fourth week it is stopped and the inhaled steroids used on their own, on a continuous basis. The tablet steroids are best taken as a single dose, and preferably before breakfast, to minimize the risk of any side effects.

Remembering to take the treatments

If an inhaled steroid has been prescribed, your biggest problem will be remembering to take it regularly. The best plan is to take the treatment less frequently, but with more puffs. Four puffs of Becotide taken twice a day are as effective as two puffs taken four times a day. And one puff of Becloforte gives a dose equivalent to five puffs of Becotide. Tablet steroids are best taken all at once, before breakfast.

B2 *nedocromil* ✳

This has been developed very recently as an anti-inflammatory agent which does not contain steroids. It is not used to reverse an attack but to prevent attacks by regular daily use. It is believed to act by preventing the release of chemical mediators from the mast and basophil cells and by blocking the release into the airway tissues of the inflammatory eosinophil cells.

It aims to be a first-line defence against challenges such as cold air and polluted air, as well as the allergic triggers such as house dust mite and pollens. In common with the inhaled steroids it can take a week or more of regular use to become effective.

Nedocromil was introduced as recently as 1986 into the hospitals, and a year later into general practice; in common with all drugs when they first appear on the market, it is, at the time of writing, being used for adults rather than for children. There is at present no known reason on grounds of safety why children should not be given it. The possible side effects appear to be confined to a mild headache or feeling of nausea in some patients, but these symptoms soon disappear.

It is prescribed under the brand name Tilade and is delivered from a metered-dose pressurized aerosol, taken usually as two puffs twice daily, with a maximum of eight puffs a day.

B3 *sodium cromoglycate (Intal)* ✳

This is not a bronchodilator but a preventive medicine which has two ways of acting: it stabilizes the mast cells, and this means that they are less likely to release their chemical messengers when faced with a challenge; it also reduces 'hyper-responsiveness' in the airways when irritants are present and, in particular, frustrates the invasion of white cells into the airway tissues, the eosinophils and neutrophils. The name 'Intal' is a shorthand for 'interferes with allergy'.

Intal cannot reverse an attack the way a bronchodilator or a high dose of tablet steroid does, but is used to prevent attacks, especially where the triggers are allergic or connected with exercise. These forms of asthma are common in children; about forty per cent of children with moderately severe asthma are controlled on Intal without the need for inhaled steroids.

There are no serious side effects. Some people get a dry throat, which is not due to 'thrush' (as is sometimes the case with steroids) and which can be relieved with a glass of water. The only snag is that Intal has to be taken three to four times a day, every day.

Intal is taken either as a powder from a capsule dispensed by a 'Spinhaler' or as a metered dose from an aerosol inhaler (in a choice of two strengths). Intal is often used in conjunction with a metered-dose bronchodilator, which is taken first.

How Intal was discovered

The late Dr Roger Altounyan was employed by a drug company to organize trials of compounds related to 'khellin'. This was the active part of a plant, Ammi visnage, used in biblical times as a bronchodilator. Dr Altounyan distrusted animal experiments, believing that 'the only thing a guinea pig has in common with man is that neither wags a tail'; he tested the compounds on himself, a severe asthmatic. After many trials he realized that he should be testing it not as a bronchodilator (for which purpose Intal proved ineffective) but as a shield against allergic asthma.

The second problem was to discover a means of delivering the drug in a large enough dose straight to the airways. Dr Altounyan recalled his war years sitting behind the propeller at the controls of a Spitfire fighter; he then developed the Spinhaler which enables the patient to draw in the powder by a sharp intake of breath.

Nowadays it can cost up to £50 million to develop and test a new drug before it is released for general use. No fewer than sixty drug companies have tried to find a compound similar to Intal, and all have failed. This helps to explain why radically new breakthroughs in drug treatment are rare and why improvements mostly take the form of better administration rather than radically new discoveries.

B4 *Ketotifen (Zaditen)* ✳

This is another preventive medicine, much prescribed on the Continent and aimed mainly at allergic (extrinsic) asthma. It is especially effective in children. It probably acts in the same way as the other preventive drugs, by inhibiting one of the mediators which recruit white blood cells, in particular P.A.F., which recruits eosinophils. In this way it can reduce 'twitchiness' in the breathing tubes, especially if the treatment is on a daily basis and continuous. It is not a bronchodilator and will not relieve an attack already under way.

Ketotifen is prescribed under the brand name Zaditen and is taken by mouth as a 1 mg capsule or tablet, or as a sweet syrup. The usual dose is 1 mg in the morning and the same again in the evening. It is not available as an inhaler. Side effects are limited: it makes some patients sleepy or dizzy in the first days of treatment, but this reaction disappears after a few days. During this time, car driving and alcohol should be avoided.

Group C: 'Acute savers' ◢
Bronchodilators and steroids

In a severe attack the aim is to deal at the same time with spasm of the airway muscles and with the inflammation, using the highest dose that can be tolerated. When a general practitioner visits an asthmatic at home in an acute attack, he will check that the available bronchodilator has been taken correctly. If this has not worked he will either use a nebulizer (to supply a high dose of salbutamol or terbutaline) or inject hydrocortisone or provide a course of prednisolone tablets. Until quite recently an injection of aminophylline would have been his first choice, but this method is used less commonly nowadays.

If there is no marked improvement despite these treatments, then he is likely to refer the patient to a hospital where staff trained to deal with such an emergency can devote the time necessary to bring the attack under control, using additional treatments if needed.

If a patient is liable to suffer these severe attacks, the doctor may provide an 'acute saver' to be used at the patient's discretion: either a nebulizer with a supply of bronchodilator or, more commonly, a course of prednisolone tablets, with instructions on how to check whether they have brought the attack under control.

Other medicines
Medicines in combination

Doctors approve of drugs used in combination, but they do not approve of drugs in which the combination is fixed in advance by the manufacturer. Some of these drugs have been used for many years (such as Franol) and, if a patient finds them to be effective and possessing no undue side effects, then a doctor will be reluctant to change. Others are quite new, designed to overcome some disadvantage in the master component, and these are judged on their merits.

BROVON: This is the combination that kept many of us going until the modern adrenaline derivatives were developed. It is delivered from a bulb-operated aerosol inhaler and consists of adrenaline (as a bronchodilator) and papaverine (an opiate to damp down the excitement caused by the adrenaline). It is very effective at relieving spasm and adrenaline is the only drug so far discovered that will prevent a breakdown of the epithelial lining of the airways when under attack. But adrenaline is not selective and leads to nervous excitement if swallowed.

FRANOL: This is a tablet which contains ephedrine and theophylline as bronchodilators and a sedative, phenobarbitone, to damp down the nervous agitation caused by the other two. Ephedrine is unsuitable for the elderly because it can adversely affect bladder emptying, and sedatives are potentially dangerous in people with severe asthma.

TEDRAL: Similar to Franol, without the sedative.

RYBARVIN: This a concoction of non-selective bronchodilators (atropine and adrenaline) and sedatives (papaverine and benzocaine).

DUOVENT: This is a combination of a selective bronchodilator (Fenoterol) and ipratropium, the anti-cholinergic drug derived from atropine. The idea is that these two in combination will produce a greater bronchodilation than either used separately.

VENTIDE: This is a combination of salbutamol (bronchodilator) and beclomethasone (steroid) in an inhaler. The aim is to open the airway with the first so that the second has greater effect. However, it could result in an excessive dose of steroid. To get round this, doctors can prescribe salbutamol separately – but in this case the formulation would seem to lose its purpose.

However, it is useful for patients who simply cannot remember to take inhaled steroid on a regular basis.

INTAL CO: This contains both sodium cromoglycate (Intal) and isoprenaline. The isoprenaline (a bronchodilator) is introduced to reverse the transient spasm which some patients experience when they inhale a dry powder which is not a bronchodilator. It also widens the scope of Intal. This combination is not much liked by doctors because isoprenaline is a non-specific relaxant and could stimulate the heart as well.

Medicines that are not appropriate

Patients receive bad as well as good advice and may be under the temptation, perhaps following advice from friends or neighbours, to search in the medicine cupboard for a remedy that might at first sight seem to be appropriate but which is not recommended by physicians for treating asthma, and which may even be harmful.

Antihistamines have to be given in very large doses to have any effect in asthma; and at these doses they may produce drowsiness, a lack of concentration and, particularly in children, nightmares. Their use with children is confined to the management of hay fever; non-sedating antihistamines are used for this purpose, as we shall see in Chapter Eight.

Cough mixtures are designed to decrease the cough reflex and are based on codeine; they will not relieve an asthmatic cough. Since this is especially a problem with asthmatic children, the appropriate measures are discussed in Chapter Five on asthma in children.

Mucolytics are designed to help a patient cough up mucus. They do not work in asthma. If there is a copious discharge of mucus, this probably indicates the need for the preventive use of inhaled steroids to damp down the inflammatory response and discharge from the mucus glands.

Sleeping tablets might seem to be a good idea when there is recurring asthma at night. They are definitely not suitable when a patient is liable to severe attacks, because in those circumstances every ounce of energy is needed to keep on forcing the breath in and out of the lungs. Even in mild asthma, sleeping tablets may be dangerous because it can be hard to predict whether the asthma will remain mild.

Are antibiotics a suitable treatment?

If a sample of patients were asked whether they find that antibiotics help them to control their asthma, most would reply that they believed they are of benefit; and many GPs prescribe antibiotics for asthmatics. The antibiotic most commonly prescribed is amoxycillin, a capsule to be taken three times a day for a full course of ten days. Any shorter course might encourage resistant bacteria to flourish.

The scientists mostly take a different view. They agree that attacks of asthma may be triggered by head colds, sore throats and (less commonly) influenza. But these infections are mainly due to viruses, and antibiotics are powerless against viruses, so there is no point in prescribing them. Furthermore the production of phlegm in asthma, however copious, does not necessarily mean that there is a chest infection. The asthma is mimicking an infection and the phlegm usually consists not of viruses or bacteria but of mucus and dead cells resulting from the inflammation.

Why then do chronic asthmatic patients believe that antibiotics can help reduce the severity or frequency of the asthma? Are we simply deluded? One reason is that in older people the asthma is often mixed with a bronchitic infection, and it is hard to separate them from each other. Another reason is that viruses can be followed by 'secondary invaders'; these are bacteria which can descend to the chest and which can be overwhelmed by a course of antibiotics. Recent research seems to support this view. This has shown that invading bacteria can damage the linings of the air passages and expose the nerves which lie beneath them so that they react to the irritants which arrive with each breath. The bacteria may also set in train the inflammatory response. However, the new technique of 'lavage', collecting mucus from asthmatic airways by washing it away using volunteers, has revealed that bacteria are rarely found in the mucus. It follows that antibiotics are generally unnecessary, especially in childhood asthma. When they are prescribed, they are used in addition to the bronchodilators and steroids and not as a substitution for them.

The role of oxygen

When an acutely ill asthmatic is admitted to hospital, oxygen is likely to be given, since the level of oxygen in the blood is likely to be low. Oxygen is often given by the ambulance crew who take the patient to hospital – and a great relief this is, as I can testify. Should oxygen be kept in the home? Physicians do not usually recommend this: it is a dangerously flammable material, and it may be used excessively so that a patient comes to depend on it.

A closer look at inhalers

Since asthma is mostly triggered when the asthmatic inhales allergens or irritants, it is not surprising that inhalation is also the best way of delivering the medicines used as the first line of defence. When taken by the inhaled route, the medicine is directed straight to where it is needed: the air passages. This means that only a tiny dose is needed to achieve its purpose and, as a result, side effects are reduced to a minimum. Not all the spray reaches the airways, but the part which is swallowed is itself so small that it causes no upsets unless the patient is extremely sensitive to the particular drug or is using the device far too often.

In the comparatively rare case in which most of the airways are so badly plugged with mucus that the spray cannot reach them, then the medicine has to be taken by way of a tablet, syrup or suppository. In a very severe attack an injection may be needed.

In this section we will look at the principles underlying the use of inhalers. A list of the brands in common use is given in Appendix E, with an indication as to which forms are available at the time of writing.

There are three ways in which a medicine can be inhaled:

as an aerosol spray:	as a dry powder:	as a solution:
(bulb inhaler)	Spinhaler	nebulizer
metered-dose inhaler	Rotahaler	
pressurized inhaler plus spacer	Diskhaler Turbohaler	
Autohaler		

The bulb inhaler is no longer widely used, but I have included it because it illustrates how a drug in solution can be turned into a fine spray. When it was introduced in the 1930s it was a great advance because until then patients were given either ephedrine as a tablet, resulting in nervous agitation, or adrenaline by injection by a doctor. By squeezing the bulb, a jet of air could be passed over a thin tube and so draw up the medicine in solution and at the same time produce a vapour, in much the same way that a carburettor in a car produces petrol vapour. The disadvantages were that the glass tubes became blocked, the dose varied with the squeeze and many droplets were probably too large to reach the smaller airways.

I METERED-DOSE AEROSOL INHALER

The aim is to produce a single measured dose in the form of a fine spray. The medicine is suspended in a liquid propellant (freon) inside a pressurized container. When the valve is opened, the propellant forces the mixture out at great speed, emerging as a cloud of fine particles which hit the back of the throat at about thirty miles an hour. At this stage the mixture is made up of propellant, lubricant and a small proportion of medicine. The metering chamber then refills in about thirty seconds and the inhaler is ready for a second puff. The freon gas is used because of its safety, though I have met a family who were concerned because they believed their teenage son had become addicted to it. A small minority of asthmatics can be irritated by the gas and the lubricants; this can cause spasm, but is immediately reversed if it

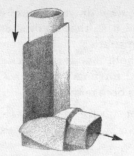

Fig 6

is a bronchodilator which is being delivered. It is more likely to cause wheeziness if it is a steroid that is being propelled, and a bronchodilator should be taken beforehand. (Some people are worried that aerosols are making holes in the earth's ozone layer and letting in a dangerous amount of ultra-violet light. Some kinds of aerosols may in due course be banned, but will be replaced by more acceptable propellants. If you are concerned about this problem, you can use a dry powder inhaler instead.)

Metered-dose inhalers may be said to have transformed the treatment of asthma since the first one, the 'Medihaler', was introduced, in the mid-1960s. The aerosol form is used to deliver not only the adrenaline derivatives but also Intal and the steroids. The main disadvantage of this method is that an effective dose is provided only when the device is used properly and this does require good co-ordination between squeezing the canister and the intake of breath. Always make sure that the way you are using the inhaler has been checked by a doctor.

1 It is best to use the inhaler standing up, with the head tipped back slightly.

2 Remove the cover and shake the inhaler vigorously in order to mix the medicine with the propellant.

3 Holding the inhaler between thumb and forefinger, breathe out gently, not so fully as to provoke a cough but with the aim of emptying your lungs of most of the air you feel inside them.

4 Immediately place the mouthpiece in the mouth and close the lips tightly round it so that no drug escapes. Start to inhale, slowly and deeply; just after you have started, press the canister quite hard – use both hands if necessary. This is done by squeezing thumb and forefinger together. Continue to breathe in until a full breath has been taken.

5 Hold your breath for about ten seconds, or as long as is comfortable, to make sure you do not expel the medicine you have just taken in.

6 Before taking a second puff, allow half a minute to pass before squeezing again. This will give the metering chamber time to refill.

7 Replace the cap on the mouthpiece.

It is not easy to remember the names of the medicines, especially when short of breath or in the early hours of the morning. The colours on the plastic actuator case help: it is worth remembering that Ventolin is blue, Becotide 50 is light beige, Becotide 100 is brown and Becloforte a maroon red. These colours can be hard to see in a low light, so I cut a nick in the mouthpiece of the blue inhaler since this is the one needed to relieve breathlessness as it occurs.

All too often the inhaler is found to be out of action, either because it has been mislaid or because it is empty. At night, when needed to relieve the 3 a.m. 'morning dip', it seems to have disappeared into the bedclothes. During the day, a quick change of clothes may result in leaving home without it. Old hands at this game make sure that they practise good housekeeping, checking each week where the inhalers are and ensuring that they are well charged. I use a letter scale to tell me just how much solution remains inside. Another trick is to remove the metal canister and place it in water: if it sinks, it is full; if it floats flat, it is empty; and if it rests suspended at an angle, then it is one-quarter full. It is prudent to leave inhalers in a number of places: in the briefcase or overnight bag; in the glove compartment of the car or in a drawer at the office. Some doctors initially prescribe half a dozen inhalers for this reason. They are best kept at room temperature

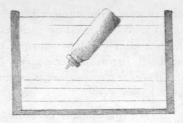

Fig 7

before use. Empty inhalers should be thrown away and replenishments obtained in good time. At night, the inhaler can be placed on the bedside table or attached to the bedpost by a loop of string passed through it.

2 SPACERS

These have been designed to overcome two of the problems that many people encounter with the metered-dose aerosol inhaler. The first is that young children, and the aged or arthritic, have difficulty in squeezing the device strongly or in timing the squeeze so as to coincide with taking in a breath. The second drawback is that the high-speed jet hits the back of the throat in a way which may be uncomfortable and inefficient.

Spacers are fixed to the inhaler and receive the aerosol spray in a small collapsible sleeve (Bricanyl) which can be carried in the pocket, or in a large plastic canister (the Nebuhaler and the Volumatic) which is quite large and cumbersome. The result is that you can breathe in normally, without worrying about timing, and you do not receive a sudden jet of medicine in the mouth. As a result, less medicine is swallowed or lost around the mouth, and a greater proportion reaches the air passages. There is also less risk of a dry throat or a fungal infection (Thrush or candidiasis).

The spacers, particularly the larger ones, allow time for the propellant to evaporate away from the tiny particles of the drug; this gives them a smaller size so that they can penetrate further into airways. Some asthmatics believe that by filling the spacer with a large number of puffs they will increase the dose taken with each puff. What happens, however, is that more drug is

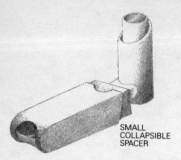
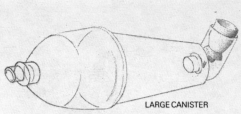

SMALL
COLLAPSIBLE
SPACER

LARGE CANISTER

Figs 8 and 9

deposited on the inside; a single puff, taken in and then repeated, is the best way.

The best technique is to hold the spacer horizontally when you breathe in the mist. Children can be taught how to use the device when it is empty and so get used to it; the valve makes a funny noise which appeals to them. Spacers are rather large to carry around and are found to be most useful for the night and morning doses.

Spacers can be obtained on prescription. The large canisters (Nebuhaler and Volumatic) can also be bought from the chemist without prescription, and cost about £5.

	collapsible pocket spacers	larger canisters
bronchodilators	Bricanyl	Nebuhaler: Bricanyl
		Volumatic: Ventolin
steroids	Pulmicort	Nebuhaler: Pulmicort
		Volumatic: Becotide
		and Becloforte

3 THE AUTO-INHALER

This has been designed so that the aerosol is fired when a breath is drawn in – so that no co-ordination is needed. The Aerolin inhaler dispenses salbutamol (in the same dose per puff as the conventional aerosol inhaler), by means of a spring which is released by inhalation and which is reset when the lid is closed after use.

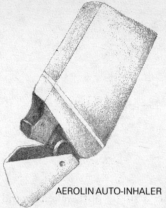

AEROLIN AUTO-INHALER

Fig 10

4 DRY POWDER INHALERS

In these inhalers the medicine is in the form of a powder which is delivered when there is a sharp indrawing of breath. In the older versions the patient inserts a capsule containing the powder into the inhaler and then punctures the capsule by twisting or squeezing the device. This releases the powder and the patient simply breathes inwards, without any need for co-ordination. The Spinhaler is so called because it incorporates a propeller to create turbulence.

There are additional advantages. Dry powder inhalers are easier to use if the hands are arthritic; you know how many doses remain, and you can take a second dose immediately. An advantage with children is that these inhalers do not lend themselves to playing squirts at school! One disadvantage is that in very severe asthma the patient may not have enough breath to take in the dose.

Single-dose dry powder inhalers are available as follows:

	Spinhaler	Rotahaler
sodium cromoglycate	Intal	
salbutamol		Ventolin
Beclomethasone diproprionate		Becotide

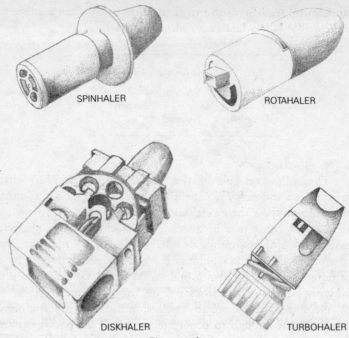

SPINHALER

ROTAHALER

DISKHALER

TURBOHALER

Figs 13 and 14

It is a disadvantage of the single-dose inhalers that they have to be reloaded on each occasion that they are used. In 1988 multi-dose dry powder inhalers made their appearance. The Diskhaler dispenses the powder from a disk which consists of eight blisters, each containing a single dose. When all eight doses have been taken, the disk is easily replaced.

The Turbohaler also uses a rotating disk. When twisted this collects a tiny amount of pure drug from a reservoir, and the drug is drawn upwards through spiral tubes which disperse the particles, the motive power being a sharp indrawing of breath. There are no carriers to act as irritants, and this also means that 200 doses can be stored in a space no bigger than the capsule used for a single dose in a conventional powder inhaler. At present this is available only for dispensing Bricanyl (a bronchodilator). It is likely that Pulmicort (an inhaled steroid) will soon be available as well. Clinical trials have shown that most patients can manage to use the device even when their asthma is severe.

	Diskhaler	Turbohaler
salbutamol	Ventolin	
terbutaline		Bricanyl
beclomethasone	Becotide	

5 NEBULIZERS

The old pocket bulb inhaler was a kind of nebulizer: when you squeezed the bulb, it expelled the medicine as a fine mist. Nebulizers produce their very fine mist by using compressed air which draws the liquid medicine from a chamber by negative pressure upwards and outwards into a mask or mouthpiece. The air, which is filtered, is compressed by an electric pump or by a foot pump like the one used to inflate car tyres. The foot pump is hard work when you have to keep going for ten minutes.

Nebulizers have three advantages: in the more efficient ones, the mist is fine enough to penetrate the small air passages even when they are partially obstructed; the device needs no co-ordination of breathing; and a large dose can be delivered. You breathe in when you wish to, and this can be a great advantage when you are very short of breath.

Most of the drugs in common use can be nebulized, with the exception of the theophyllines. The drugs are provided in solution in ampoules or small bottles. Among the bronchodilators Ventolin, Bricanyl, Berotec, Bronchodil and Atrovent can be delivered by nebulizer. Among the preventive medicines, Intal and Becotide can be taken in this way.

The great majority of asthmatics can control their asthma with a conventional inhaler. If co-ordination is poor, they can use a spacer. So it may be asked, why are nebulizers prescribed? There are three kinds of patient who may benefit from using a nebulizer:

• Regular use of the protective medicine Intal can make a big difference to children with asthma. Below the age of four or five, though, they find it hard to use any of the pocket inhalers, so

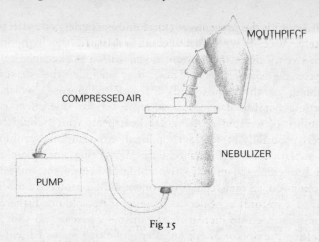

MOUTHPIECE

COMPRESSED AIR

NEBULIZER

PUMP

Fig 15

Intal is often given from a nebulizer. Becotide can also be given in this way. In children under eighteen months, nebulizers can aggravate the asthma and are not normally used outside hospital.

• A very small number of people whose asthma is both severe and chronic find that they do not respond to the small doses of bronchodilator obtained from pocket inhalers; they are given a nebulizer to deliver the drug, 2–4 times daily. Doctors try to reduce the need for this by prescribing preventive medicines.

• Severe acute attacks of asthma respond very well to bronchodilators given from a nebulizer. This treatment is not confined to hospitals and GPs may use a nebulizer in the home; they are sometimes available in ambulances, and some patients have a nebulizer to use in a crisis, in accordance with the plan that has been worked out with their GPs. This plan should cover: (a) the warning signals that indicate the need for a nebulizer; (b) how much medicine to put in the nebulizer; and (c) what to do after using the nebulizer. It is essential that any patient who has been recommended a nebulizer should know how to set it up, how it acts and how to keep it clean.

Doctors are divided in their opinions about the regular use of nebulizers; many prefer to confine their use to dealing with an acute phase or administering a preventive medicine to young children. With the preventives (Intal and Becotide), side effects are unlikely. With the nebulized bronchodilators, the high dosage (often twenty times the amount taken with a pocket inhaler) can increase the side effects. These may include 'the shakes', a trembling of the hands and a feeling of unease, which are unsettling but not dangerous. A more serious side effect is the possibility of a rapid or irregular heartbeat, which could be of concern especially in an elderly patient. An additional problem is that a high dose of bronchodilator may bring immediate relief from bronchial spasm but do nothing to reduce the underlying inflammation, so that regular treatment with a protective medicine (Intal or a steroid) is neglected. If relief is not obtained, there is a temptation to go on increasing the dose – whereas you should be consulting the doctor about an alternative treatment. Patients can put too much faith in their nebulizers.

Nebulizers are not available on prescription and they cost about £70–100 (ninety per cent of the cost is for the compressed-air pump), so it is not a good plan to rush out and buy one unless a doctor has recommended it and has explained how to use it. The model chosen should be capable of delivering droplets as small as three microns. If used each day, a record of peak flow should be kept, as will be explained in the next chapter. The unit should be kept clean at all times and be serviced once a year. Some hospitals have a home nebulizer service for this purpose.

Chapter Four

ADJUSTING TREATMENT TO SUIT THE ILLNESS

How bad is the asthma?

Picture yourself in the doctor's consulting room – not as the patient but as the doctor! Each asthmatic patient has a different story to tell, in language which is far removed from the precise terms of the medical schools. 'Would you say that the attacks are mild or severe?' One patient will describe as mild symptoms which another will consider to be severe. Some agreed definitions are needed.

The doctor will also need to know whether the asthma takes place occasionally (i.e., is episodic) or is more or less continuous (i.e., is chronic). It will also be of interest to the doctor whether the attacks are worse at night or during the day.

In their research programmes, Fisons Pharmaceuticals rely heavily on patients' descriptions of their asthma, before and after testing a new remedy. The company use the table opposite to enable patients to record the severity of attacks.

For ease of reference we may translate these scales, which refer to daytime asthma, into the four rather crude categories that appear in the right-hand column of the table.

We also need to be able to describe the breathing difficulties which take place at night. In mild asthma it is very probable that the patient will wake up in the morning feeling wheezy, or that sleep will be interrupted; a puff of bronchodilator is sufficient to restore the breathing to its usual level. In very severe asthma, sleep is impossible.

In any asthmatic the severity may change from one season to another, or from one week to the next. In my recollection, asthma in childhood used to be episodic and mild – except during scale

0	no symptoms of wheeze or breathlessness	
1	occasional wheeze or breathlessness, which is easily reversed with an inhaled bronchodilator	**episodic & mild**
2	wheeziness or shortage of breath occurs most of the time but does not interfere with the usual activities at home or at work	**chronic & mild**
3	wheeziness or shortage of breath occurs most of the time and there is some interference with the usual activities	**chronic & severe**
4	asthma very bad. Could not go to school/work or carry out the usual household duties	**acute & severe**

the height of the pollen season when it became severe and persistent. From late middle age onwards it became chronic and it is especially likely to be severe when the weather is unstable.

Patients with chronic asthma are particularly at risk that their asthma may deteriorate into a *very severe* attack, sometimes known as *Status asthmaticus*. The patient may experience one or more of the following very distressing symptoms:

• Breathing is in short, sharp gasps. These are difficult to control so that the advice to 'keep calm' may be misplaced (unless it is applied to the onlookers!).

• Wheezing ceases. So little air is able to move in and out that the chest is silent. *This is a danger signal*.

• The patient is in bed or on a chair, from which he or she can rise only with the greatest difficulty.

• The patient feels weak and trembling; there is profuse sweating and a feverish feeling.

• It is impossible for the patient to speak more than a few words at a time or to explain what his urgent needs are; these may include a desire to visit the lavatory to attend to a loosening of the bowels, or to have a drink of water.

• The patient feels exhausted; after a time the feeling of lassitude may pass into a loss of consciousness – this is *a very dangerous phase*, since if coma follows the doctor will now have to deal with a situation of great danger.

• There may be a blueness about the nails and lips. This indicates a severe lack of oxygen and *immediate medical assistance is needed*. Loss of consciousness and coma may follow.

All the above descriptions assume either that there has been no medical treatment or that the treatment has been ineffective. They have the disadvantage that they do not trace the progress of the attack over time or provide any accurate measurement of the lung capacity.

Asthmatics think they know just how bad their asthma is by the feeling of tightness in their chests. But this can be misleading. Some mornings, when I wake, the asthma may seem severe but then subside after the merest whiff from the inhaler. A few days later, this situation seems to be repeated until I stir about – and then find I am very short of breath. When resting in bed or in a chair, very little oxygen is required; the absence of wheeze does not mean that the lungs are free from obstruction. What is needed is some way of measuring this obstruction in relation to a scale of severity. This is now available in the form of a simple **peak flow meter**.

The invaluable peak flow meter

If your breathing tubes have become narrowed or partially blocked, you will find it difficult to blow out hard. Your 'peak flow' will be diminished. A peak flow meter is a device which registers this peak flow on a scale. You blow into the mouthpiece as hard as you can; this pushes a needle along the scale, and the value is expressed in litres per minute. It is very easy to operate.

1 Stand up, remove any false teeth and hold the device level.

2 Take in a full breath – through the mouth or the nose – and fill out your chest until it will go no further (to 'total lung capacity').

3 While holding your breath, close your lips tightly, making sure that the meter's cursor is at the bottom.

4 Blow out as fast and as hard as you can through the mouthpiece and not at all through the nose. There is no need to empty your lungs.

5 On a meter designed for adults, the needle will stop somewhere between 60 and 800. On a meter made for children, the scale runs from 30 to 370.

6 Repeat the exercise twice; note all the readings and choose the *highest* (not the average) reading. This is usually the first of the readings.

What is measured?

You have just measured your P.E.F.R., the maximum peak expiratory flow rate, in litres per minute. A chart is provided with the device which shows what non-asthmatics achieve, on average, according to sex, height and age – for example, a male of my age and height should reach 560 litres per minute. This is my **predicted peak flow**. As a chronic asthmatic, however, my P.E.F.R. never rises above 320 in daytime, even when my chest feels quite clear. This is my **best or usual peak flow**. The dips in the flow tend to be assessed as percentage drops below this **best** level.

The chart provided for children relates peak flow to height rather than to age or sex – for example, ninety-five per cent of non-asthmatic children with a height of 140 cm (4'6") will achieve a P.E.F.R. of between 250 and 400 litres per minute. At a height of 180 cm (6'), this will rise to between 450 and 600 litres per minute. Children can use a peak flow meter from the age of five or six.

The mini-Wright Peak Flow Meter is light and strong and measures to an accuracy which is quite acceptable to doctors. It is not at present available on a National Health Service prescription, but it may be issued by a hospital, donated from a charitable source, bought from the chemist, or obtained at maker's cost plus postage from the Asthma Society. Specify whether a child's or an adult version is required. Another light plastic meter is supplied by Vitalograph Ltd (the manufacturers' addresses can be found under Useful Addresses at the back of this book). Cost varies in the range of £7–9 when bought through the Asthma Society.

The diary card

The symptoms described relevant to one moment only are not nearly as useful as those recorded over a period of time. This is why patients or their parents are increasingly being asked to keep a daily record of peak flow for a limited time, for example over the period until the next consultation. It may also prove useful as a guide for times when the patient is at special risk from seasonal or other factors, such as staying in a new environment.

What is recorded will depend on the card that is used. The example given opposite is based on cards used by two London hospitals; it enables the following information to be recorded using severity scales:

- changes in symptoms

- activity

- peak flow meter readings

- the medicines used over the 24 hours

- comments such as (a) saw doctor; (b) absent from work/school; (c) any infection; (d) away from home; (e) any dramatic change in the weather (e.g. mist, thunder, a wet spell) that may have contributed.

It takes only a few minutes to fill in the daily column, but the reward could be a marked improvement in treatment if the card is carefully studied by your doctor. It provides a common ground of

THE DIARY CARD
NAME.............MONTH.............YEAR........

Date			1	2	3	4	5	6	7
last night	good night	0							
	slept well, slightly wheezy	1							
	woken 2–3 a.m.	2							
	bad: mostly awake	3							
wheeze last	none	0							
night	little	1							
	moderately bad	2							
	severe	3							
cough last	none	0							
night	occasional	1							
	frequent	2							
activity	normal	0							
today	can run a little	1							
	can only walk	2							
	off school or work	3							
peak flow	(best of 3 blows)								
	before a.m. medicine								
	before p.m. medicine								
medication	took as prescribed?								
	took extra doses?								
	took different med?								
	if so, which?								
additional	runny nose?								
info	itchy/puffy eyes?								
	weather change?								
	sore throat?								
	other illness?								
	saw the doctor?								
	travel away from home?								
Queries for the doctor									

information which all can share; it could also encourage the less confident to ask such questions as: 'You tell me that the medicine will enable me to lead a normal life, but doctor, is it really normal to wake up at 3 a.m. with a wheezy chest, two or three times a week?'

There is an added bonus! It is all too easy to forget to take the medicine that has been prescribed; this lapse has to be recorded on the card. Most asthmatics under-treat their asthma, and this may be corrected if a diary is kept. Make copies of the diary on page 99, try keeping the diary for a few weeks, and then show it to your general practitioner for his comments. If he tells you that you have been wasting your time, then you will at least have the private satisfaction of taking a contrary view.

Interpreting the results

The dialogue between the patient and the doctor will be more fruitful if they share an understanding of what the diary can reveal. These diary cards are now issued by many chest physicians and at asthma clinics in health centres. The following four examples show how daily records, transferred to a simple graph, can reveal the kind of asthma that has to be treated. When the treatment is under way, they show whether or not it is succeeding in restoring the peak flow to the best possible level for the patient concerned.

(1) The 'morning dipper' (Fig 16a)

Many asthmatics report that their worst symptoms are experienced when they wake up in the small hours of the morning. This is known, not surprisingly, as 'the early morning dip'. The dip in peak flow will persist until the patient rises to begin the day's activities and takes the medicines. So night-time asthma is recorded as an 'a.m.' reading and daytime asthma as a 'p.m.' reading: confusing at first, but quite logical.

Figure 16a shows a regular fall in a.m. peak flow compared with the early evening reading which will register the daytime peak flow (asthma tends to improve during the day). The vertical

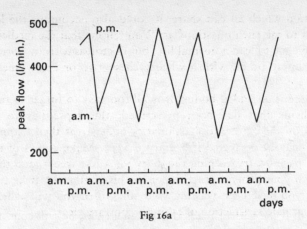

Fig 16a

scale is used to record the peak flow reading in litres per minute. The horizontal line divides into morning and evening readings.

The aim of treatment will be to reduce the fall in peak flow and also to shift the average between a.m. and p.m. a little higher. Even normal people show a small reduction in peak flow at night, but in asthmatics it may drop by at least fifteen per cent, and in some cases by as much as fifty per cent. It is an astonishing fact that lung function, as measured by peak flow, can drop significantly, to about half that of normal, before some patients become aware that they have restricted breathing.

The morning reading is taken before the medicines are administered, i.e. at the time you wake with early morning wheeze or (if there has been no night asthma) before breakfast.

(2) The 'slow slider' (Fig 16b)

Patients get used to their symptoms and tolerate them, so they do not notice the slow deterioration until it is too late and find themselves in hospital after a most unnerving attack. If, on the other hand, we adopted the practice of keeping a diary of peak flow readings at times when we know we will be especially at risk (for example, in September when the children start again at school and spread infections around) then such a crisis might be

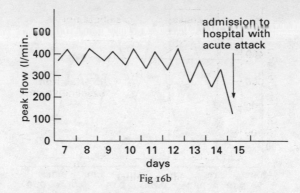

Fig 16b

avoided. If the patient reads the warning signs, he will consult his doctor, or change the treatment, in time to prevent the acute attack.

(3) *Wheezy after exercise* (Fig 16c)

When the asthmatic turns up at the 5 p.m. surgery, he or she may show no sign of asthma. In order to confirm the diagnosis, the doctor may ask the patient to take vigorous exercise, having first taken a 'baseline' peak flow reading. The peak flow is recorded every minute after the exercise for fifteen minutes and a bronchodilator is given to restore the normal function. The peak flow is measured; the patient runs round the surgery for six minutes; then peak flow readings are taken.

Over eighty per cent of asthmatics will show a fall in peak flow of at least fifteen per cent within ten minutes of stopping the exercise. The rapid improvement after a bronchodilator has been used is another indicator that it is asthma.

(4) *The 'brittle asthmatic'* (Fig 16d)

Peak flow readings over time can also be used to assess what kind of asthma is being experienced. Some patients experience fluctuations in their asthma which are so variable and unpredictable that they are described as having asthma which is 'brittle'.

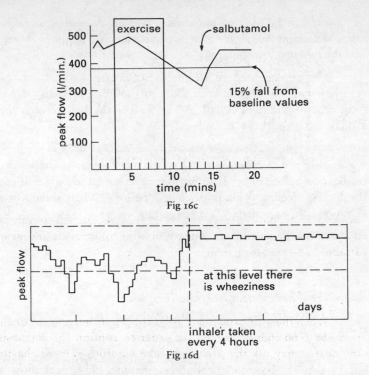

Fig 16c

Fig 16d

What tends to happen is that peak flow falls dramatically over a few minutes and is then reversed by a couple of puffs from the bronchodilator inhaler, but this effect does not last.

This reading from a typically 'brittle' asthmatic may suggest to the doctor that the patient is not using the inhaler regularly but only when symptoms occur. If it is used four times a day, at intervals of four hours, then the asthma may become less variable and the peak flow may rise above the level at which wheeziness is experienced. Volmax is now available for longer-acting Ventolin treatment.

The uses to which a peak flow meter can be put may be summarized as follows:

• By measuring the response to a bronchodilator, it can help the doctor confirm, or set aside, a diagnosis of asthma.

• It can be used to pinpoint a trigger. A reading is taken when the suspected trigger is present and again when it is absent, and the two results compared.

• It can be used to decide whether the asthma can be reversed with a bronchodilator alone or whether it needs steroid treatment in addition. A fall of half below the best level is the kind of indicator that is considered.

• Asthma may worsen gradually; regular peak flow readings will enable you to seek help, or step up the dosage, or change the medication before rather than during the acute attack which is the result of a decline. This is discussed below, 'When should you summon help immediately?', on page 113.

• Peak flow readings will provide an objective assessment of a child's asthma for parents.

How does the doctor choose the treatments?

We have studied the illness and its many triggers. We have surveyed the remedies, including the medicines which are used nowadays, and we have looked at the various ways in which they can be taken. We then considered how the severity of the illness could be assessed by observing the symptoms and by measuring the peak flow. Peak flow readings can also be used to decide whether or not the treatment has been effective.

Let us now return to the surgery and put ourselves in the place of the doctor. How does he decide what treatment to prescribe? First of all, there must be a detailed case-history. This will reveal whether the asthma is episodic (occasional) or persistent; whether it is usually mild or quite often severe. A note will be made as to whether there is wheezing or coughing at night, after exercise, or after meals. The patient may be asked to take home a peak flow meter and enter readings on a diary card, and to return to the surgery after a set time for a further assessment. 'What the doctor needs to know' is elaborated in Appendix B on page 201.

The doctor decides on a treatment plan.

By way of illustration, I invite you to consider four fairly typical plans, which relate to four different kinds of asthma. It should be borne in mind that all treatment is on a trial-and-error basis, that doctors vary in the way they approach medication, and that they also have to take into account factors (such as home circumstances, age, experience, other illnesses) which cannot be included in these brief notes.

The aim of the simple case-histories that follow is to provide some insight into the way the doctor will choose a plan of medication which distinguishes between 'the sword' and 'the shield'.

relieving drugs	the sword	⚡	bronchodilators
preventing drugs	the shield	✳	anti-inflammatory and anti-allergic drugs

This distinction is observed in the cases which follow, but it should be remembered that when the bronchodilators are used regularly three or four times a day, they also act as preventers to a limited extent.

The cases are illustrated by actual histories (with the names changed), but the treatments could apply in principle to any age group above infancy. Later, we shall be studying asthma in children and dealing with some of the special problems that arise in that situation. This will be followed by a chapter on adult asthma.

A. *Mild episodic asthma*

Patient: 'I just wheeze sometimes.'

Peter, a young man in his early thirties, had mild, episodic asthma as a child, but fortunately grew out of it in his teens. By the time he was in his twenties he had no symptoms of wheeze or breathlessness. He has recently become very health-conscious and keen to keep fit and avoid 'middle-age flab'. He has now cut down on animal fats, has a high-fibre diet, eats lots of fruit, fish and vegetables and has taken up marathon running. It is hard luck that, with all that sensible attention to diet, he finds that the running makes him very short of breath after about ten minutes. He asks the doctor what he should do.

DIAGNOSIS: episodic asthma, in this case brought on by exercise. Mainly due to bronchial spasm which will be reversed with a bronchodilator

TREATMENT:

🖊 take inhaled bronchodilator when needed, as a reliever

✳ take bronchodilator ten minutes before exercise; and keep the inhaler handy, to be used when wheezy

✳ as an alternative, or in addition, take Intal before the exercise

B. Moderate persistent asthma

Parent: 'She gets asthma quite often now, at least four or five times a week. They are not severe attacks but we feel that the asthma is not being properly controlled.'

Mary, aged five, fair haired and blue eyed, is a very lively child, advanced for her age. She had eczema as an infant, but this responded well to treatment with hydrocortisone cream. When she joined a play group she tended to get short of breath when racing round the hall. Quite recently she has started to waken her parents at night with fits of coughing and a slight shortage of breath. This is causing distress to all concerned.

It is also of concern that Mary frequently has head colds, and these are invariably followed by a spell of wheeziness, again not severe but persistent.

DIAGNOSIS: the wheeziness after exercise, the coughing at

at night and the wheeziness after a virus infection all add up to typical signs of asthma. In particular the persistence of the attacks and the night asthma (which could be confirmed by taking peak flow readings before breakfast) call for regular preventive treatment.

TREATMENT:

⊞ take Intal 3–4 times a day every day, even when there are no symptoms. In adults, and in children who are not controlled on Intal, take an inhaled steroid 2–4 times a day, every day, regardless of symptoms

⬆ take a bronchodilator as necessary and half an hour before play or exercise, from an inhaler

If the night coughing persists, then additional treatment may be needed (see 'night cough' in 'The principles of management', page 133).

After a year, stop the regular treatment to see if the asthma can be controlled on the 'reliever' (the bronchodilator) alone.

Many doctors nowadays start with the inhaled steroid as a preventer because it will deal with any inflammation and need be taken only twice a day.

With young children, mothers find that a bronchodilator given as a syrup is sometimes the only way they can persuade the child to take the medicine, and the only effective way when the breathing tubes are tight.

C. Acute severe asthma

'Doctor, can you come and see me. As you can hear . . .
I am very . . . short of . . . breath . . . and the inhaler does
not seem to be . . . having any . . . effect.'

Sarah, aged thirty-five, developed hay fever when a
teenager and this coincided with the examination months
of June and July. The hay fever has remained but is well
controlled on a steroid nasal spray (Beconase), provided
she remembers to start taking it before the pollen season

begins. Quite suddenly in June 1985 she started to wake at night with coughing and wheezing – not every night but three or four times a week. By August, the symptoms had disappeared. All this was bearable – but one night in July 1986 she found herself severely short of breath and, in a state of alarm, rang the doctor.

DIAGNOSIS: an acute and severe attack. The normally mild asthma moved into a second-phase attack, and this will not respond to a bronchodilator given from a pocket inhaler.

TREATMENT: before the doctor arrives
✒ Much depends on what is available in the home. Ideally the patient should immediately take a high dose of tablet steroids (e.g. 8 × 5mg tablets of Prednisolone) If a nebulizer is available, with a bronchodilator, this should be used at once

TREATMENT: when the doctor comes
✒ The doctor will assess the seriousness of the attack and he will probably rely on a nebulized bronchodilator in a high dose
✒ plus steroid in a high dose, either nebulised, or as tablets of Prednisolone, or as an intravenous injection of hydrocortisone. If an ambulance is called, then oxygen may be given on the way to the hospital

TREATMENT: a plan for the future
The doctor will make sure that the patient is provided with a plan for ongoing treatment and also a 'crisis plan' to be used if there is another severe attack
⊞ The doctor will make sure that the patient keeps on the high dose of tablet steroids for at least ten days, and after that will prescribe inhaled steroid to be taken night and morning at first in a high dosage
In addition, the way the patient uses the bronchodilator from an inhaler (dry powder or metered-dose aerosol inhaler) will be checked

D. Severe persistent asthma

Patient: 'I seem to wheeze most of the time and asthma wakes me at night at least three times a week. At times the attacks are difficult to control with a bronchodilator.'

Anthony, aged ten, a quiet child, has had asthma and eczema since he was eighteen months old. He was referred to the outpatients department of the Paediatric Unit at the hospital and they recommended that he should have a nebulizer at home, for administering salbutamol (a broncho-dilator). Rarely do twenty-four hours pass without him wheezing and coughing, and he has had many bad nights and a lot of time away from school. In his case the triggers were all too numerous: not only the allergic triggers of pollen in the hay season, and cats, but also non-allergic triggers such as exercise, virus infections (i.e. head colds) and laughter. His mother relied on giving salbutamol (Ventolin) through the nebulizer when the attacks became really bad but did not think that anything more could be done. One evening the attack was so bad that he was brought to the surgery, with a peak flow of 80.

DIAGNOSIS: the asthma is both severe and persistent; the breathing tubes are hyper-responsive and react to quite small triggers. This means that there is inflammation in the airways as well as muscle spasm. The peak flow is probably depressed all the time, but it may well be possible to restore it to a normal level, given the correct treatment.

TREATMENT:
✒ Steroid tablets are taken in a high dose for a limited period (Prednisolone) and then, when the asthma is stabilized, the treatment is changed to
▣ an inhaled steroid taken regularly, night and morning, even when there are no symptoms (e.g. Becotide, Becloforte or Pul-micort)

⊞   The inhaled bronchodilator will continue to be used before exercise (or Intal as an alternative), also night and morning; and it can be used to relieve wheeziness when required

🖋 In addition, some doctors will provide the mother with an emergency treatment: tablets of oral steroid (Prednisolone) to be taken if there is a severe acute attack in advance of any emergency visit by or to the doctor

It is unlikely that troublesome night asthma will persist if the above treatments are carried out. ⊞ A slow-release bronchodilator in tablet form may be tried at night as an additional measure.

ASSESSMENT: the mother may be lent a peak flow meter and asked to keep a diary for a couple of weeks, then to report back to the surgery so that the doctor can check whether treatment has worked as expected.

What you should do if things go wrong

The above case-histories have been examined from the point of view of the doctor; they have been included in order to give some insight into the way the treatments are adjusted to suit the frequency and severity of the asthma. The doctor's prescription is designed to last for some time, perhaps for a year or longer if repeats are indicated.

The patient or parent may have to make day-to-day adjustments if the asthma is episodic or not well controlled. The checklist which follows reviews some of the more common situations and suggests the appropriate action. Written by a general practitioner for his asthmatic patients it has been slightly changed to suit this format.

WHEN SHOULD YOU SEE THE DOCTOR?

As soon as you think you are not controlling the asthma: do not wait until you have to call the doctor in an emergency. This is explained in the next section.

YOUR INHALER DOES NOT BRING RELIEF.

Take it along to your doctor; he will check that you are using it properly. He may suggest a different kind of inhaler.

YOUR TABLETS OR SYRUP DO NOT WORK VERY WELL.

You may manage better with an inhaler: see your doctor.

YOUR WHEEZES GET WORSE WHEN YOU HAVE A COLD.

Increase the dosage from the bronchodilator by taking more frequent puffs while the cold lasts.

YOU WHEEZE WHEN YOU TAKE EXERCISE.

Use your bronchodilator beforehand: an hour if you use tablets or a syrup; ten minutes if you use an inhaler.

YOU WHEEZE WHEN YOU GO OUT INTO THE COLD.

Use your bronchodilator inhaler about ten minutes before you go out (whether or not you are wheezing).

YOU WHEEZE WHEN YOU PAY A VISIT ...

... because there is something at the place to which you are allergic. Take a dose of your bronchodilator about ten minutes before you arrive and repeat as often as needed. Better still, if your doctor has provided you with a prescription for steroid tablets, take 10 mg every day for the duration of the visit. Some children can be very well protected against this kind of allergic risk by being put on a course of Intal.

YOU OFTEN WAKE AT NIGHT WITH WHEEZING.

As far as children are concerned, this is discussed in Chapter Five, 'The principles of management,' on page 133. You should consult your doctor, who will prescribe either an inhaled steroid to dampen down both day and night asthma or a slow-release bronchodilator which will last for the whole night.

THE EFFECT OF YOUR INHALER DOES NOT ACT LONG ENOUGH,

Sometimes you will find that you want to use your inhaler more often than has been prescribed, because the doses seem to be becoming less and less effective. This is a WARNING SIGN that the asthma attack is becoming more severe. *If the effect of a dose is lasting three hours or less* you should call the doctor straight away. If you have been given tablet steroids as an emergency treatment, take the full emergency dose straight away, even though you have made an arrangement to see the doctor. When he checks the situation, he may decide that you need preventive treatment as well as the relieving bronchodilator, on a regular basis.

YOU HAVE BECOME A 'SLOW SLIDER'.

That is to say:

• your wheezing has been getting worse over a number of days

• you have a morning wheeze which is taking longer and longer to clear

• the attacks are lasting longer and are hard to check with full doses of the drugs you normally take

You may need to take a full course of tablet steroids to make you better. Your doctor may allow you to keep a limited supply of these, to use according to the instructions he gave you previously. This will be especially useful if you spend time away from home or tend to have severe attacks. Then consult your doctor and tell him you have used up your emergency supply.

YOU HAVE A SUDDEN SEVERE ATTACK OF WHEEZING . . .

. . . that is not relieved by the bronchodilator. You should carry out the **Crisis plan** that has been agreed in advance with your doctor. This may consist in taking a further dose of an inhaled bronchodilator every ten minutes for half an hour. By 'dose' is meant two puffs from an aerosol inhaler or one puff from a powder Rotacap inhaler. If this works, then revert to a dose every four hours. If it does not work, call the doctor. He may have provided tablet steroids to use in an emergency in which case take the full emergency dose straight away, in addition to the bronchodilator.

If you are too wheezy to move, a doctor should be called immediately. These guidelines will be elaborated in the next section.

When should you summon help immediately?

In some ways this is the most important section in the whole book: a patient's life may depend on making the right decision. The answer is surprisingly simple:

> Call the doctor as soon as you feel that the attack is slipping out of control, after taking the medicines you have been given to relieve it.

In other words, let the experts decide whether or not the attack is dangerous. They have had years of training in dealing with just such an emergency, and they have the right equipment. You, the patient or parent, have had no formal training – and in any case you are too upset to act in a wholly rational way. The doctor is paid to do this work, through your health service.

It is quite rare for a general practitioner to be called out at night-time: far from resenting a summons, your doctor will be only too pleased to deal with a situation which may carry a high risk. As one junior hospital doctor told me: 'I enjoy treating asthmatics: you give them enormous relief, with minimal effort.' That is of course only half the story: how to avoid the next crisis is a more complex problem.

It happened, on the very day I wrote the first draft of this section, that I developed a severe asthmatic attack, away from home, and had to make this all-important decision. The circumstances are fresh in my mind, so I will relate them to you.

After typing the draft, I packed hurriedly (forgetting to include the peak flow meter) and drove into the country. It was a glorious morning in early autumn, the end of a spell of fine weather. As I arrived, at lunchtime, the clouds rolled over, humidity rose and the temperature dropped dramatically. I had been a little wheezier than usual, but a couple of puffs from my inhaler seemed to clear this. Having no peak flow meter at hand, I could not check the real state of my airways.

Later in the day a delicious evening meal was provided, with wine. Just at the end of the meal an acute attack of asthma developed. I climbed the stairs slowly to my room to retrieve the 'crisis' pack. At the top of the stairs the extra effort had made the attack very severe indeed, with breaths coming in short and (fortunately) loud gasps and speech almost impossible. I managed to take the special medicines (a high dose of bronchodilator and a high dose of tablet steroids). At the same time my friend called the local G.P. He had to return to his surgery to collect a nebulizer, and arrived half an hour later.

By this time the peak flow had recovered to 200 litres/minute. After ten minutes of inhalation of a nebulized dose of bronchodilator it had reached only 250, so my friend drove me to the hospital, where the usual measurements were taken (peak flow, pulse, blood pressure) and the usual soundings with stethoscope and X-ray picture. However, no more medicine was needed. The combined effect of my crisis plan and the doctor's nebulizer had brought this quite dangerous attack under control. By the following day, peak flow was back to my usual daytime level of 350.

This was a typical two-stage attack, the first being mild and the second one, following six hours later, much more severe. I told the doctor who attended about the book I was writing and he commented: 'Do please tell your readers that asthma can kill and that they should observe three golden rules.'

• If you are in any doubt as to your ability to cope, ask someone to call your doctor, or dial 999 for an ambulance. Do not delay: get them to telephone at once, at the very moment when it becomes clear that this is no run-of-the-mill, easily reversible episode.

• Immediately take the medicine you have available, in accordance with whatever crisis plan you have worked out in advance with your doctor, or in the light of your own experience.

• In a crisis most patients under-treat their asthma, so sometimes deaths take place which could have been avoided. Take the full dose at once and not in stages.

This accords with the advice now given by chest physicians. To quote Dr Philip Snashall: 'It is the illness which is dangerous, not the medicines.'

When your doctor receives your phone call, he will need to decide whether to attend personally, summon an ambulance, or take both actions. Having discovered the age and sex of the patient, he will need to be given some idea about the patient's appearance: posture; colour of face, lips and nails; rate of breathing. He will need to know what medicines have been taken to deal with the attack. If the patient has been nebulized without improvement, then a hospital visit may be indicated.

There are further lessons to be learnt from my trip to the country.

• Always take your peak flow meter with you. The ways in which it can help assess the severity of an attack are described above, page 96.

• A severe attack may take place when you are out of reach of a doctor, when the car breaks down, say, or in a foreign country or on a walking holiday. Make sure your 'crisis plan' is fully worked out in advance, when you are well.

• If, during a severe attack, you find that you can speak only a few words, gesture for a pencil and paper to be brought, so as to be able to convey your needs.

We will return to this theme when looking at asthma in children (on page 121), but at this stage it is sufficient to note some of the warning signs that the asthma is seriously out of control.

What are the warning signs?

For the majority of asthmatics, the illness is mild and the attacks of wheeziness are easily reversed with an inhaler designed to relieve spasm. Nevertheless, all asthmatics and their families, and teachers with asthmatic children in their classes, should be aware of the warning signs, the indications that the asthma is out of control and that a telephone call should be made to the doctor without delay.

You should call the doctor if any of these occurs:

• The inhaler has no effect; if there is a crisis plan for additional treatment, this will also have failed to reverse the attack.

• Peak flow has dropped to half its normal best reading in daytime (assuming that a peak flow meter is available and that the normal level for the patient has been established).

• Breathing is in short, sharp gasps which cannot be controlled by the patient as to depth or frequency. If the wheezing ceases this is a real danger signal: there is so little air going in and out that the chest is silent.

• The patient is on a bed or chair from which he or she can rise only with the greatest difficulty.

• The patient can utter only a few words, forced out between gasps.

• There is a blueness about the lips and tongue, or the fingernails. This is another signal of real danger: the next stage would be sinking into unconsciousness, so you should dial 999 for an ambulance as well as calling your doctor.

While waiting for the doctor or ambulance to arrive, the carers should avoid making any signs of fuss or panic or anger. These will add to the patient's fears and make the breathing even worse. Onlookers should reassure the patient that medical help is on its way. The patient should be allowed to adopt the position which he or she prefers – and this is likely to be one of the postures illustrated in the next section. The patient will be very thirsty, and a glass of water should be provided. Any physical movement should be avoided if possible because this would call on the depleted reserves of energy; if essential (to attend to a loosening of the bowels), it should be assisted.

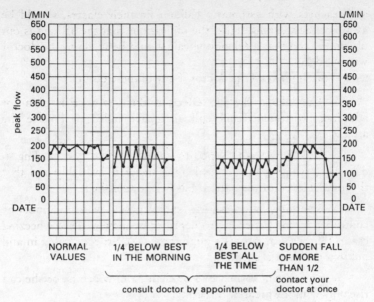

Fig 17. What to look for in your child's peak flow patterns

Peak flow readings can offer guidance

Danger levels will vary from one patient to another. Each asthmatic has a normal day- or night-time peak flow level which is called the 'best level'; this will be lower than the levels achieved by non-asthmatics. What is important is not the absolute value but the percentage drop from the best level.

Armed with the kind of charts reproduced here (by courtesy of Fisons Ltd) the patient can establish with the doctor when to call by appointment and when to call as a matter of immediate urgency. It will be seen that falls of one-quarter below the best readings either in the early morning ('early dip') or all the time are signs that a change of treatment is needed. If there is a sudden fall of more than one-half, then you should call the doctor at once. The peak flow readings will supplement the subjective assessment of symptoms already described.

This may be easier to understand when expressed as a table.

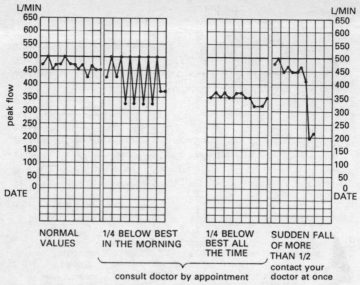

Fig 18. What to look for in your own peak flow patterns

	ADULT	CHILD	
best level (say)	500	200	the yardstick *
¼ below best	375	150	consult doctor
½ below best	250	100	seek help straight away
approaching ¾ below best	150	60	danger level

With experience, asthmatics can learn how to deal with the quarter below and the half below normal levels as soon as they occur.

It is our aim in the next two chapters to help the reader achieve this kind of expertise, not simply by reading this book but also by working out a plan with the paediatrician, chest physician or family doctor. Having established the crisis level at which additional medication is needed, it might be a good idea to write it on the label of the meter. If the asthma is so severe and chronic that the best level is always below, say, 200, then the rules suggested above will have to be modified.

* This will vary from one patient to another.

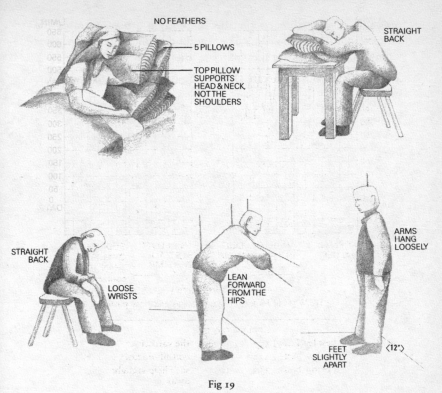

NO FEATHERS

5 PILLOWS

TOP PILLOW
SUPPORTS
HEAD & NECK,
NOT THE
SHOULDERS

STRAIGHT
BACK

STRAIGHT
BACK

LOOSE
WRISTS

LEAN
FORWARD
FROM THE
HIPS

ARMS
HANG
LOOSELY

FEET
SLIGHTLY
APART

⟨12"⟩

Fig 19

Posture during an attack

In a severe attack the patient tends to adopt the posture which seems to him to be most helpful. During a talk given to our branch of the Asthma Society, the Superintendent Physiotherapist at the Brompton Hospital in London explained that some postures, especially the sitting ones, are preferred when there is a severe attack:

1 Take the bronchodilator as prescribed.

2 Aim to breathe with minimum effort, so as to make the greatest use of the limited supply of oxygen.

3 Aim to relax the upper part of the chest and to relieve the

pressure of the stomach on the diaphragm (this separates the lungs from the stomach). The method will depend on your situation. Five ways are shown in the illustration.

4 Breathe at your own rate. It may be easier to do this with the mouth open.

Chapter Five

LIVING WITH AN ASTHMATIC CHILD

A series of challenges

The parents' first reaction to a diagnosis that their child has asthma is likely to be one of shock and uncertainty. What does the future hold in store? Is the child going to suffer a lifetime of illness? In reality, if the asthma is typical of that of the majority, it will be mild, occasional and easily managed with simple treatments, which will allow the child to lead a full and normal life. Even so, the parents will still have to adjust to those sudden and alarming attacks of breathlessness, to the paroxysms of night coughing and to the child's silent appeals for help when there seems to be no immediate improvement. Much depends on what picture is formed of the illness.

Living with asthma in the family presents many challenges. Not the least of these is that it is hard to judge the seriousness of the attack and to know when you need to summon a doctor. There are worries about the medicines, and there may be difficulty in persuading the child to take them. There are countless anxieties as to what may be causing the asthma and, perhaps associated with this, a feeling of guilt that not enough is being done to remove the causes.

The parents are not likely to receive much help from family and friends if these people have not had experience of the illness. Asthma tends either to be dismissed as a trivial complaint, easily reversed with modern medicines, or to be seen as a nervous condition, made worse by 'over-protection'. The parents are advised by those around them to wait until the child grows out of the asthma, and in the meantime simply put up with it.

The family doctor will be able to set the record straight and provide that badly needed reassurance. But the average doctor is under pressure, consultations can be hurried affairs and can leave the parents as confused as ever. So they tend to feel isolated and threatened. Friendships are put to the test and the marriage itself may come under strain through the stress of coping with the illness.

It may be of some comfort to learn that asthma is one of the commonest illnesses in childhood. It affects one child in ten and is responsible, more than any other illness, for keeping children away from school. It is not therefore surprising that self-help groups have been formed, which enable parents to share their experiences with one another. At the time of writing, the Asthma Society has 160 branches, spread around the country; its work is discussed in Chapter Eleven.

Children themselves, with their enormous vitality, are pretty resilient. They come to accept asthma as the normal way of life, the only one known to them. The attacks may be terrifying, their outcome seemingly uncertain – but they are soon forgotten when breathing becomes normal again. Children learn to accept the constraints that asthma imposes, and adapting to it presents a challenge, along with all the other challenges they meet as they grow up.

How can the doctor tell it is asthma?

The fact that 'asthma' as a diagnosis tends to alarm parents has led to a silent conspiracy on the part of some doctors to avoid this diagnosis and to refer instead to rather meaningless phrases such as 'wheezy bronchitis' or a 'wheezy chest'. This concealment of the truth may have the unfortunate result that the parents will suspect that something is being hidden from them, that the illness is more severe than is really the case. It can also lead to inappropriate and useless treatments. In a study, which is now famous in medical circles which was carried out in Newcastle-upon-Tyne in 1983, all the children aged seven were examined in a large area of the city. It was found that out of 176 children who were wheezy only twenty-one had been told that they had asthma.

How does a doctor decide that a child has asthma? If the patient appears in the surgery in the afternoon, the symptoms may have disappeared, so the doctor has to rely largely on the parents' own observations. It is helpful if these have been sorted out before the consultation takes place. He is likely to ask if any relatives have or have had asthma, hay fever or eczema. Wheezing is the commonest sign, but some asthmatics do not wheeze. There are five questions in particular which, if the answer is a definite 'yes', will show the doctor that there is asthma.

1 Do the wheeziness and tightness get worse at night, especially around 3–4 a.m.? Is there coughing at night?

2 Does the wheeziness get worse following exercise? If the answer is a definite 'yes', then this is a certain sign of asthma. If there is no clear answer, the child may be asked to run up and down the street, or use an exercise bicycle, with readings of peak flow taken before and after to see if this has diminished as a result of the exercise.

3 Does the wheeziness disappear within a few minutes of taking a couple of puffs from an inhaler containing a bronchodilator?

4 Does the wheeziness often follow a virus infection such as a head cold?

5 Has the child missed odd days from school, from time to time? If the answer to any of these questions is 'yes', then the child probably has asthma.

The questions that parents ask

I have already dealt in an earlier chapter (on page 28) with questions concerning asthma and heredity. Asthma, eczema, hay-fever, urticaria and migraine tend to run in families. The chances that a child will develop an 'atopic' illness of one kind or another are about twelve per cent if neither parent has atopy, twenty per cent if one parent has atopic symptoms, and forty-five per cent if these have appeared in both parents. About forty per cent of asthmatic children also develop eczema, an illness which is beyond the scope of this book but which will be covered in the list of addresses (see page 212). This leads logically to our first question.

SHOULD WE HAVE CHILDREN?

The fact that there is a relative on both sides of the family with severe asthma does not mean that the children will have asthma which is severe. It is more likely to be mild and therefore easy to manage. If one child already has asthma, there can be no guarantee that the next will be free – but the chances are in favour of this being so.

IS MARITAL ENGINEERING A GOOD IDEA?

In order to reduce the load of challenges which the newborn child has to face, every asthma-sensitive and ultra-sensible couple may decide to avoid times of birth which will coincide with the peak pollen season (June and July) or the peak mould season (early autumn); or the peak time for house dust mites (autumn and early winter). That at least is the suggestion of Dr John Warner, an allergist at the Brompton Hospital. This restriction would fortunately leave clear the favourite month for births – March.

If a mother has been told that she has a higher-than-average level of IgE antibody in the blood and a lower-than-average level of the 'T-cells' which suppress the antibodies, what can she do? Breast feeding may help. In the critical first six months allergens and irritants should be avoided wherever possible: no animals, total war on the house dust mite and the ban on cigarettes continued.

DOES ASTHMA PRESENT PROBLEMS IN PREGNANCY?

With good medical care women with asthma have no more trouble during labour than women without asthma. About a third of pregnant women find their asthma improves during pregnancy, a third do not notice any change and a third find their asthma gets rather worse. Any improvement will be due to an increase in the production of steroid by the mother's adrenal glands. It will not necessarily happen in the second pregnancy.

Women have to breathe more when they are pregnant, but only to a small extent compared with the tenfold increase in breathing which takes place during vigorous exercise.

The pregnancy itself is unlikely to be affected by having asthma, and the risk of a severe attack during labour itself is extremely low because the adrenal glands pour out cortisone and adrenaline into the blood. Smoking should of course be avoided during pregnancy anyway.

CAN THE DRUGS USED IN ASTHMA AFFECT PREGNANCY?

The adrenaline derivatives, such as salbutamol and terbutaline, are sometimes used by obstetricians to try to prevent premature labour, but in very high doses; when used to treat asthma in much lower doses, they do not have this effect – and this is in any case a debatable result: many obstetricians do not believe that these drugs have any effect on the pregnancy even in the high doses. Aminophylline has been found to be safe in pregnancy. Sodium chromoglycate appears to be safe in every condition. This leaves the steroids which, if given in tablet form, could reach the baby in small amounts and possibly reduce the baby's own steroid production.

The reverse may be true: some of the sedatives used in pregnancy should not be given to mothers who can be asthmatic, and some of the drugs used to induce labour can cause a tightening of the airways.

IS VACCINATION SAFE?

Whooping cough is particularly dangerous for asthmatic children, with its prolonged fits of racking cough. These can cause a child to vomit and, in extreme circumstances, to stop breathing. Against this, and for all the other routine immunizations plus those carried out before travelling abroad, children with asthma can be vaccinated even when an attack is in progress. This is also the case with the other forms of allergy. The measles vaccine may not be suitable for a child who suffers an extreme reaction to eggs, if sick from a fever, or if on a course of steroid tablets; for these and similar precautions consult your doctor.

ARE BOYS AND GIRLS EQUALLY LIKELY TO DEVELOP ASTHMA?

It is a remarkable and so far unexplained fact that, in childhood asthma, boys outnumber girls by two to one, up to the age of thirteen years. After that, the girls catch up with the boys. In the more severe forms, boys predominate. It is not known why this should be so.

Hormonal factors affecting asthma are also seen in the menstrual cycle. In women with asthma it may get worse before the cycle and then improve during the early part of the cycle. It can be treated with progesterone.

DO CHILDREN CHANGE THEIR SENSITIVITIES?

The commonest cause of wheezing that lasts for more than a few days is an infection of the nose, and often of the throat as well, in the form of a cold. This is especially so in the first three years of life, when wheezing and coughing are almost always brought on by viral infections. It seems that not only are antibiotics useless; there are no adequate vaccines either – and in any case the child must develop its own immunity.

In older children, allergy also plays an important part; in fact, half of all children will show up as positive on a skin test to at least one allergen, even though only ten per cent of children develop asthma. Food intolerance may play a part in some children, especially to milk and eggs. From then until puberty, the house dust mite is the main allergic trigger. As a result of a continuous exposure to house dust, the children come to tolerate it to some extent; and then the various pollens and moulds tend to take over as the most common allergic triggers. It is more difficult to acquire a tolerance of these because they come and go on a seasonal basis.

Non-allergic causes, especially the virus infections we have mentioned, exercise and cigarette smoke, can provoke attacks at any age.

CAN ASTHMA AFFECT GROWTH?

In some children, especially those with chronic asthma, there is a delay in the spurt in growth which takes place immediately after puberty. The delay may be as long as two years. Such children tend to be shorter and lighter; this may be disconcerting to the child, who sees siblings and peers forging ahead. Fortunately, the delay is temporary and the asthmatic child then catches up and achieves his or her full stature.

IS CHEST DEFORMITY COMMON?

Chest deformity used to be a common feature in children with severe chronic asthma. Nowadays this is rare because this type of asthma can be controlled with inhaled steroids which, even if taken daily, do not suppress growth. The existence of chest deformity can be taken as a sign of inappropriate treatment. Fortunately it can be reversed after a year or two.

DO CHILDREN GROW OUT OF ASTHMA?

The incidence of asthma diminishes by halves. It is most common in the first five years of life. In half of these children, the asthma subsides or becomes trivial. Puberty is another time when half of those still asthmatic show a marked improvement, with many losing their symptoms. Many grow out of their asthma in adolescence. But asthma can return five or ten years later. It is very hard to predict who will be the fortunate ones, except to say that those with severe asthma at any stage are the least likely to improve. It follows that parents and children should face this possibility and consider it when choosing a career.

There is not much that parents or doctors can do to alter the long-term outlook, with a single exception: tobacco smoke should be avoided because it may do more harm to a child's lungs than any other irritant.

SHOULD WE MOVE HOUSE?

Parents sometimes worry that where they live may be responsible for the asthma. They hear tales of people 'who felt so much better when they went to live at so-and-so'. It can happen that when the family moves house the child's asthma does improve for a time. But this tends not to be maintained, and the stress of moving could prove to have been unnecessary. If allergy to grasses is a major factor, then it may be better to live in a city, preferably not too close to a main entry route, with its extra load of car exhaust, or to an underground or main trunk sewer, with an extra load of dampness. In the context of damp, a well-built modern house may be more suitable than an old house which has been poorly built.

It would be unwise to assume that, if you take a holiday by the sea or up a mountain, you can leave all the medicines behind. Children may meet new triggers when on holiday and need to take their medicines with them, including the 'crisis' pack.

SHOULD WE CONSIDER A SPECIAL SCHOOL?

It is possible to send your child to a special boarding school, the Pilgrim's School near Brighton, which takes children with severe and persistent asthma. No fees are paid by parents (local authorities are asked to contribute). Far from being over-protected at the school the children manage through expert care to cast aside what may have been a crippling disability and learn to excel in all the activities that healthy children enjoy. Children with severe asthma who are very unhappy at their present school, or who are unable to cope at home, benefit greatly from being able to mix and compete with other children on equal terms.

The principles of management
Managing asthma in infants

When a baby enters the world following its sheltered life in the womb, it has to adapt to a place where many decisions have to be made. It has to distinguish between things which are good for it (such as food) and things which are bad for it (such as germs and toxic substances). It develops an immune system whereby injurious particles are attacked, surrounded and over-whelmed, while harmless and beneficial substances are accepted and tolerated. Some babies decide that particles entering their airways are harmful, and thus become wheezy or develop a night cough, even though the particles could easily be cleared through the wafting of mucus up and out of the airways. But the most common trigger for asthma in infants is not an allergen, such as house dust, but a virus infection.

Asthma in infants has proved difficult to treat. In about forty per cent of cases they respond to nebulized ipratropium bromide (Atrovent). But the other drugs, when nebulized, seem only to increase the wheeze and lower the peak flow in the first ten minutes or so. This may have something to do with the solutions, which in themselves can cause bronchoconstriction, because they are weak and acidic and contain preservatives. It also relates to the way the infants receive the spray; it has recently been shown that the drugs can be more effective if delivered from a much cheaper device: a spacer (Nebuhaler or Volumatic) fitted with a face mask, which acts as a re-breathing chamber with the valve kept open. It may also have something to do with particle size, and this varies according to the type of nebulizer used. It is likely that most of the dose of nebulized steroid is taken in in the first five minutes, and prolonged dosage (which increases the intake of the carrier) may not be needed. All these ideas need further testing but do look promising.

Fortunately, symptoms in babies are usually mild and time is the best healer. About eighty per cent of wheezy infants grow out of their symptoms by the time they are ten years old. If the symptoms are severe or persistent or seem to be increasing in severity, then a visit to the hospital is indicated, especially as asthma in infants is often missed and treated inappropriately. As children develop, they can manage an increasing variety of treatments which can be tested from the age of about twelve months. In the meantime, parents fall back on syrups to deliver the bronchodilator and use the nebulizer as a standby in the more severe cases.

Managing asthma in older children

The principles are the same as when managing asthma in adults: parents must start a dialogue with the doctor which will enable the treatments to be used effectively, with a 'crisis' plan worked out in advance should the asthma suddenly get worse. The special problems that arise with children relate to their inability to report on their illness and to take the medicines on their own initiative.

We have already studied the possible ways of reducing the triggers.

The points that need emphasizing where children are concerned are that the bedroom should be kept as free as possible from house dust and animals, that smoking should be banned and that, when parties and special occasions are being planned, the preparations should be kept in a low key, since attacks can be brought on by excitement.

What are the warning signs? It is always easier to deal with an attack in the early stages, and any of the following signs may be taken as an indication, in a child prone to asthma, that an attack is under way:

- a persistent cough

- a runny, then a stuffed-up nose

- irritability

- a disinclination to eat

- breathlessness following any increase in physical activity such as climbing the stairs

- a tendency to become easily tired and lethargic

- wheeziness

- some difficulty in talking

In the classroom the teacher may detect a lack of concentration, and the child may sit at the desk with hunched shoulders.

In early childhood, asthma often appears not as wheezing but as fits of coughing, most commonly at night or when waking in the morning or after exercise. If there is wheezing, it may take place only after contact with an animal, or there may even be no obvious trigger. Younger children are especially likely to be affected by house dust mite, which occurs all the year round; asthma in the pollen season is more typical of older children.

Treating asthma with medicines

In most children, asthma can be managed at home by using a variety of simple medications. As we have already seen, the choice of medicine depends on the type of asthma.

ASTHMA WHICH IS MILD AND EPISODIC

Three-quarters of children who are asthmatic have isolated attacks which respond to simple treatment with a bronchodilator. The attacks may be short or long in duration, according to the triggers which provoke them, but they are fully reversible: that is to say, the breathing returns to normal between attacks. This can be judged from the peak flow readings.

The form in which the bronchodilator is given will depend on the age of the child:

Approximate age	
infancy	nebulizer or syrup
2½ years	aerosol with spacer
4 years and upwards	dry powder inhaler
5 years and upwards	metered-dose aerosol inhaler

Slow-release tablets are also used, and may be crushed in food.

The medicines available in these forms are listed in Appendix E.

THE ATTACKS ARE INFREQUENT BUT SEVERE

Some asthmatic children have attacks which occur less frequently than, say, once a month, but they are sometimes severe. Between the attacks the children are free from wheeze and breathlessness, and peak flow readings return to normal. In these cases the inhaled bronchodilator may not be capable of reversing the attacks, even at twice the normal dose. Possible treatments include the use of a nebulizer to provide a much higher dose of bronchodilator, or a short course of steroid in tablet form, in order to restore peak flow to normal. The steroid course will run for only 10–14 days, and no permanent side effects will be experienced. If neither of these treatments is available, then the doctor should be consulted.

THE ATTACKS ARE FREQUENT BUT MILD

The attacks are mild but they are frequent and last for an extended period so that the asthma must be regarded as 'persistent', especially if peak flow readings do not return to normal in between attacks. (In the four case-studies in the previous chapter, Mary provides an example of this kind of attack.)

The persistence calls for regular preventive treatment. The medicine that is tried first is sodium cromoglycate, best known under the brand name Intal, which is effective in about half the children with persistent asthma. If this proves to be ineffective, an inhaled steroid, for example Becotide or Pulmicort, is used on a regular basis. In addition, the inhaled bronchodilator is taken as needed, and before play or exercise, as we shall see in a later section. The asthma is checked from time to time with a peak flow meter and the preventive treatment is discontinued, on a trial basis, if the peak flow returns to normal.

About half the children who have frequent attacks in childhood continue to have asthma in adult life; in a quarter, the asthma becomes mild and infrequent and another quarter grow out of it.

THE ATTACKS ARE BOTH PERSISTENT AND SEVERE

In a very small proportion of asthmatic children, perhaps under five per cent of all children with asthma, the attacks are frequent, prolonged and often severe, and the peak flow readings never reach what is normal for the age of the child. In such cases the very high responsiveness has to be damped down with anti-inflammatory medicine, taken night and morning in the form of an inhaled steroid. (An example of this condition has already been given in the case studies, that of Anthony.)

Activities have to be restricted to those which can be tolerated. There are likely to be some admissions to hospital; in between the worst episodes, a regular check at the surgery or clinic will be essential, to ensure that the best possible treatment is being given at home and is being taken in the correct way. A crisis plan, with the appropriate medicine, is essential.

The aim in treatment will be to rescue the child as rapidly as possible from the severe attack, using either steroid tablets in high dosage or a nebulized bronchodilator or both. The second aim will be to lift the whole day and night peak flow pattern to a new and higher level, by the use of the inhaled steroid, so that the pattern is closer to the normal.

In spite of their disability, even children in this severe category do manage to lead a fairly normal life and take part in outdoor activities which are moderately strenuous, so building up their phsyical, mental and moral strength.

THERE IS PERSISTENT NIGHT WHEEZE OR COUGHING

This is distressing for all concerned. The coughing may go on and on, so that everyone loses sleep. Breathlessness and coughing at night are common in asthmatic children and, if persistent, must be regarded as a sign that the asthma is at least moderately severe and that the *daytime* asthma is not being properly controlled. It will be made worse by an infection.

The doctor's first aim will be to break into the cycle, and this means a short sharp course of steroid tablets. He will also make sure that an adequate dosage of inhaled bronchodilator is administered during the day; this should also be available when needed at night. It is quite possible that the child is not using the inhaler correctly or that a spacer would provide a more effective dosage, for example, a Nebuhaler or a Volumatic.

If regular preventive medicine is not already being used, then this will be needed, in the form of an inhaled steroid, or Intal, or Zaditen, to take over when the course of tablet steroid ceases. If inhaled steroids are already being used, then the doctor may decide to increase the dose from twice to four times a day. It is possible that a slow-release bronchodilator, taken last thing at night and effective over eight hours, will help to keep night spasm at bay. This may contain salbutamol (Volmax) or terbutaline (Terbutaline SA) or theophylline (Nuelin SA, Slo-Phylline, etc.).

When to call the doctor as an emergency

I make no apology for returning to a theme which has already been treated in Chapter Four, 'When should you summon help immediately?', on page 113. In childhood asthma, it is the adult who usually has to make this decision; it is essential that he or she can interpret correctly the signs and symptoms which indicate that the attack is so severe that medical help should be sought at once.

Many parents are reluctant to call the doctor, especially at night time, though this is when the asthmatic is most often at risk. As already explained the principle to follow is very simple:

WHEN IN DOUBT SHOUT!

In other words, TELEPHONE IMMEDIATELY. The doctor will not necessarily need to visit, especially if you have worked out a **crisis plan** in advance and have the appropriate medicines to hand. If the doctor is likely to be delayed, he may decide to call an ambulance – and you yourself should summon one by dialling 999 if you feel that not a second should be lost. When it arrives, you may wish to direct it to a hospital with which you are familiar and in this case you need to be armed with a special card, to be obtained in advance from that hospital.

The warning signs that asthma has entered a severe and possibly dangerous phase are the same in both child and adult asthma, though the measurements differ. Any one of the following symptoms may be regarded as a warning signal; in practice more than one is likely to appear at the same time.

A severe attack

• **Breathing rate.** If higher than 50 a minute in a child under five years and higher than 40 a minute in a child over five years, the attack is severe.

• **Strained breathing.** This is shown by a pulling in of chest near the neck as extra muscles are brought into play.

• **Speech difficulty.** This clearly suggests a difficulty in breathing; when the child is concentrating entirely on making each breath, then he or she will be silent.

• **Pulse rate.** This is not easy to take in such circumstances. In children over four, a rate of over 130 a minute would be considered severe.

• **Vomiting.** This is a sign that so much mucus has accumulated that vomiting is needed to clear it.

• **A sudden fall in peak flow.** If this falls to one-quarter of the normal daytime or one-quarter of the normal night-time level, the attack is a severe one. A chart illustrating this was given in the last chapter.

Danger signals

• **Exhaustion.** This is a sign that the attack is very severe. If the child becomes dazed or lapses into unconsciousness, then breathing could cease.

• **Wheezing may disappear.** This is also a sign of a very severe attack, because the child is not taking in or passing out enough breath to make any noise.

• **A bluish colour.** In light-coloured children a bluish colour may appear in the lips, mouth and nails. This is a sign that there is a serious shortage of oxygen in the blood supply – a danger signal, because the next stage will be a lapse into unconsciousness.

You may have already established which symptoms and signs call for immediate medical attention – preferably well in advance of any of the three DANGER signals appearing. When you call the doctor, you will be advised what medicines to give the child immediately, depending on what is available at the time. They are likely to be the ones indicated in Group C on page 79:

• a high dose of bronchodilator, via the most efficient means, for example through a spacer or nebulizer. A dry powder inhaler is not likely to help because it needs a strong sharp puff from the patient. When the doctor arrives, he will most probably give salbutamol or terbutaline in a nebulized dose, twenty times the dose provided by just two puffs from an aerosol metered-dose inhaler

• a high dose of tablet steroid (Prednisolone) may be indicated at the same time, as prescribed by the doctor.

Make a note of the medicines that have been taken (including especially any theophylline preparations) so that the doctor or casualty officer at the hospital will know what is needed additionally.

During and after the severe attack

Since panic is easily communicated to the child and may reinforce the attack, you must remain calm, however alarmed you may feel; there must be a complete absence of fuss. It will probably serve no useful purpose to order the child to breathe more slowly, since the rate of breathing in a severe attack is wholly automatic; instead you should explain that help is on its way and that the medicines may take a little while to bring the attack under control.

The child will adopt the posture which seems most comfortable. The aim, as explained in the last chapter, will be to let the stomach hang forward, to avoid putting pressure on the diaphragm. Avoid feather pillows and dusty cushions. There may be dehydration, due to excessive breathing through the mouth, intense sweating and sometimes vomiting. A glass of water should be at hand. If the child wishes to go to the lavatory, some assistance may be needed. Clothing should be loosened.

Immediately after the attack, the child will be exhausted and will need to rest in order to build up the store of energy that has been depleted. Unless there is a bad viral infection, however, children recover quickly, usually within a couple of days; and it is the parents who will need more time to get over the worry and tension. The doctor will explain how to adjust the treatments so that they revert to normal.

A stay in hospital

It may be prudent, while waiting for medical help to arrive, to prepare your child for a stay in hospital, and you may wish to stay with him or her in the ward for the first night, to provide reassurance in what will seem a strange and frightening environment. If your child is liable to severe attacks and has never previously been inside a hospital, a prior visit to the children's ward when well could be a good plan, so that it seems a normal and friendly place to be in.

Treatment in the hospital to deal with a severe attack is likely to include:

- a bronchodilator given through a nebulizer (terbutaline or salbutamol)

- a short course of steroids at a high dose, given as tablets or as a slow-release injection

- fluid replacement, through a 'drip'

- oxygen

Relief from the attack will not necessarily be immediate: it may take 2–8 hours to bring the attack under control. The child will probably be kept in overnight so that progress towards normality can be checked. An X-ray photograph may be taken to help confirm the diagnosis of asthma.

In the hospital, the child is the centre of attention; he or she may come home, expecting to receive the same four-star treatment. But the parent will be exhausted, keen to catch up on all the neglected chores, and worried that another hospital visit may soon be needed.

Asthma at school

Parents probably fail to realize that schoolteachers receive no training of any kind in how to cope with an asthmatic child and are denied access to the medical records, yet they are supposed to act *in loco parentis*. When there is an attack, the parent may be unobtainable; the teachers may have no idea who the family doctor is, and they are very unlikely to know what the various medicines are designed to achieve.

So the parents should not blame teachers who subscribe (out

of ignorance) to the prevailing myth that asthma is a nervous or trivial illness, or who are unaware that asthmatic children can play a full part in school activities if the medicines are taken correctly. Teachers have to act by such rules as they are given; if the parent tells them that 'the blue inhaler must be used at 2.30 p.m.', then they will be reluctant to produce it at any other time.

Because each child's asthma is different, the teachers must take guidance from the parents as to what suits that particular child. It is essential that teachers and parents should meet and talk over the treatments, with the child present, so that all agree on the right course of action. Make sure that every teacher, including those responsible for welfare and physical education, is given your instructions (in writing) as to why, how and when the medicines should be used. If this meets with resistance, then it can be backed up by a letter from the doctor to the head teacher. A very useful leaflet called 'Asthma at School' can be obtained from the Asthma Society.

It must be established that wherever the child goes, the bronchodilator goes too. It will not help if an attack takes place on a football pitch half a mile from the school and the inhaler is locked in a school cupboard. The preventive use of the inhaler *before* exercise should be made clear.

The school nurse has an important role to play, especially in teaching both child and supervising teacher how the inhaler should be used. It is possible to teach quite young children both how to cope with asthma at school and to summon help when needed. (Some school nurses say that the trouble starts when the holidays begin and daily disciplines are relaxed.) She will also be able to describe to the teachers the signs and symptoms that indicate an immediate call to a doctor or hospital is needed. Incidentally, both teachers and nurses are liable to change each year, and so the new ones should be briefed; in any case, the treatments may have changed.

Efforts are being made, for example by local branches of the Asthma Society, to set up classes in school, at which the illness can be explained to all the children. On these occasions the asthmatic children may have much to contribute to the discussions;

being asked to show those present how well they use their inhalers will help to overcome any shyness about their medication. You should make sure that the school has spare inhalers and that your notes identify which is which ('the blue one is used to relieve an attack; the brown one only for prevention').

Teachers are usually aware that they should stay with a child, during an attack or a visit to hospital, until the parent arrives. They may not be aware of the need to loosen clothing and what position the child prefers to adopt in an attack.

Games, swimming groups and physiotherapy

Exercise is not only one of the ways in which children keep healthy: it also contributes to growth. It is in dream sleep and in exercise that those hormones are released which promote normal growth. Taking part in games and sports can improve a child's self-confidence – but only if able to compete on equal terms with the other children.

Unfortunately most children with asthma become wheezy as a result of exercise – in fact this is one of the signs that doctors look for when they diagnose the illness. The typical picture is that shortage of breath takes place not during the exercise but as soon as the child pauses for a moment to rest. The attack can last for half an hour or longer.

Teachers should understand that all but the most severely asthmatic children can play a full part in physical activities such as games and sports – but only if certain procedures are followed:

• The child takes an inhaled dose of either sodium cromoglycate (Intal) or a bronchodilator (Ventolin and Bricanyl being examples) about ten minutes before the exercise starts.

• If a peak flow meter is available, this can be used to check that the breathing is up to its predicted level.

• Warm-up exercises in short bursts help to prepare the lungs for the more strenuous activity that is to follow.

• Particular care should be taken in cold or damp weather to avoid exercise which is prolonged and which (like cross country running) involves the whole body: the legs as well as the arms.

• It may be easier for an asthmatic child to cope with a position on the soccer field which involves short bursts of running rather than continual motion: in the defence rather than galloping up and down as an attacker.

• In highly competitive sports, bronchodilators may be used, but (illogically) inhaled steroids may not be used in cycle races. (Perhaps they are being confused with anabolic steroids?)

Swim Groups

Swimming is so good for asthmatic children that special Swim Groups have been formed in many parts of the country, often in association with local branches of the Asthma Society. There are very good reasons why swimming is ideal exercise for many asthmatic children:

• the body is supported by the water so that less oxygen is needed to carry out movements than in any other form of exercise

• the warm humid atmosphere of the indoor pool mimics the warm humid air that is delivered by the upper to the lower respiratory system

• the exercises can be adjusted to the child's condition, and supervision by trained instructors can be provided

• parents and non-asthmatic brothers and sisters can also join in

Some children find that chlorine can trigger an attack; some pools use ozone instead, and this too can cause wheeziness. In any case it is sensible to check with the peak flow meter that the asthma is under control before the swim and to give a preventive dose of Intal or inhaled bronchodilator twenty minutes or so beforehand. Swimming can restore sagging self-confidence. Picture a child who was described to me by a Swim Group instructor as not only severely asthmatic but also seen by those 'nearest and dearest' as a 'wimp', a born loser in every department of school life. His father in particular, a soldier who revered physical prowess, seemed to despise and reject him. However, the child decided to take up swimming; as a result he gradually grew stronger. After a couple of years he became the best swimmer in the school. In the following year, the school won the League Championship; he was now a hero to friends and family alike.

At the time of writing, the Captain of the British National Swimming Team is Adrian Moorhouse, M.B.E. He had asthma at an early age, and in his teens this interfered with games and running. A chest specialist persuaded him to persevere with swimming – which he did to such good effect that he won gold, silver and bronze medals in the Commonwealth Games, and in 1988 a gold medal at the Seoul Olympics. He has written: 'I don't think that asthma has interfered with my ambition at all because I haven't let it. I just keep on training. I suppose it made me more determined, because at school I was never going to get into the athletics or rugby team.'

Can physiotherapists help?

In children with asthma the chest muscles are well developed and stronger than in normal children, so special exercises for these muscles are not needed. But there are other ways in which the physiotherapist can help, such as teaching children how to breathe in a more relaxed way, and these are described in Chapter Two, which deals with exercise as a trigger. Very occasionally children get into problems because mucus plugs form in the airways and this can cause the lung beyond the affected area to collapse. The physiotherapist can expand this area.

Exercise should be imaginative, dynamic, interesting, enjoyable, varied and accessible, and without adverse effects, if it is to become habitual. Physiotherapists are great communicators and can help satisfy these demands.

Chapter Six

LIVING WITH ADULT ASTHMA

The changing pattern of asthma

In early adult life asthma is likely to diminish, to the extent that about eighty per cent of those whose asthma started in childhood achieve a complete recovery at this time. As they pass into middle age and beyond, half of these experience no further trouble, but half have a relapse. Asthma can start at any age, and late-onset asthma is likely to be the kind that persists.

As we grow older, the allergic triggers become less important; the non-allergic irritants, such as virus infections, dry and cold air, and pollutants, such as industrial fumes and cigarette smoke, take over as the most common immediate causes of asthma. When asthma appears for the first time in older people who have had no previous experience of it, there may be no response to the skin prick tests which reveal atopy (allergy).

In older adults, asthma tends to be non-seasonal and persistent. In many older asthmatics there is an undercurrent of wheeziness, and the peak flows achieved are below those reached by non-asthmatics of the same age and sex. As has been explained in an earlier chapter, this does not mean that the lungs are damaged, as in emphysema or chronic bronchitis. It does imply a state of permanent hyper-responsiveness, in which the breathing tubes are ready to react to quite small triggers. Since most of these are unavoidable, the older asthmatic has to rely a good deal on continuous preventive treatment with inhaled steroids, used as a shield. Adult asthma can be mixed with chronic bronchitis brought about by heavy cigarette smoking, and this creates a problem of diagnosis and treatment.

The adult asthmatic has some advantages over the child

with asthma. Adults are better able to monitor their own illness and adjust the treatment. They have more control over the environment at home. They can more easily talk to the doctor about treatment and discover what the medicines are supposed to achieve. On the debit side, asthma in adults can affect earning capacity. There is the special problem of 'occupational asthma' caused by the materials handled and adults are often affected by the ventilating and air-conditioning systems used in windowless offices. Humidifiers can accumulate asthma-provoking bacteria, moulds and pollen grains and eject them into the office atmosphere. In some offices, infections spread like wildfire; and the journey to work by public transport presents its own challenge to the chronic asthmatic.

After a time, the chronic asthmatic tends to forget what a normal airway feels like; in order to avoid undue exertion or exposure to cold air, he or she adapts life to suit the asthma on a permanent basis. In 1978 the results of a trial were reported, in which the patients' assessment of their asthma was compared with an objective assessment obtained from peak flow readings. It was found that the asthma was nearly always worse than the patient realized – the reverse of what had been generally supposed.

Recognizing the degree of severity

This has been a recurring theme in the present book. With adults, it is possible to consider the progress of an unchecked asthma attack in a way which takes into account the physiology, the symptoms and the tests available to the patient and doctor alike. This is set out in the accompanying table, which assumes either that no corrective treatment is given or that it is inappropriate. The aim of treatment is always to break into the cycle and arrest the downward slide in peak flow which could otherwise lead, very rarely, to coma and respiratory failure.

In many adults, asthma is mild and intermittent, easily reversed with an aerosol bronchodilator. In the chronic and severe form, the wheeziness persists for much of the time and intensifies if there is a drop in air-temperature, or in damp foggy weather or in the presence of a virus infection. It becomes a normal occurrence for

Type of asthma	Inflammation	Changes in the breathing tubes	Symptoms	Tests
mild, episodic	reversible	none, except muscle spasm which reverses	none between the episodes cough (may be)	peak flow returns to normal between the episodes airways narrow if given a histamine challenge and this is a sign of bronchial hyper-responsiveness (BHR)
mild, chronic	permanent	smooth muscle thickens the inner lining becomes leaky; so do mast cells inflammatory cells invade from the blood supply		
severe chronic with acute episodes	permanent	smooth muscle constricts swelling of the tissues (oedema) increased discharge of mucus →	wheeze tight chest cough (may be) breathlessness (may be)	peak flow depressed below normal readings and below the levels at which symptoms are experienced BHR increases: less histamine needed to produce a 20% drop in peak flow
danger level reached	severe	→ disorganized → very poor supply of oxygen	very rapid breathing (*status asthmaticus*) leading to coma	peak flow right down, below 70% of normal

The degrees of severity which are possible in untreated chronic asthma (adapted from A. J. Woolcock, in *European Journal of Respiratory Diseases*, Vol. 69, 1986)

It is assumed that the airways are continually exposed to an assortment of triggers which serve to reinforce the asthmatic response and that no medicines are taken.

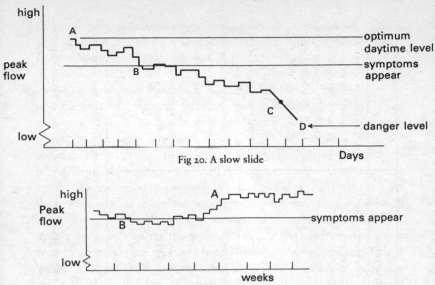

Fig 20. A slow slide

Fig 21. Successful treatment

sleep to be interrupted. In this persistent kind of asthma, the peak flow can enter a downward slide, falling below the point at which symptoms appear until the point ('C') is reached, with the reading at three-quarters of the best level achieved by the patient. It takes only a small drop when you are at 'C' to reach the danger level 'D'.

The doctor's aim when treating someone with severe chronic asthma will be to prevent the peak flow from dropping below 'B', and then to lift it to a higher level, closer to the predicted normal level 'A'.

We looked at this kind of treatment in Chapter Four when considering the case of the child. Anthony. Adult medication often proceeds along the same lines. The rate of improvement will depend on whether treatment starts at 'B', 'C' or 'D' on the severity scale shown in Fig 20.

The medicines used in adult asthma

The same medicines are used as are appropriate in child asthma: the complete range of bronchodilators and the anti-inflammatory steroids. The anti-allergic drugs (Intal and Zaditen) tend to be used less, since allergy plays a smaller part in adult compared with child asthma. Intal can be used successfully where the adult has a specific allergy, say to cats, combined with a bronchodilator.

In adults, as in children, the medicines used may seem to have become ineffective. This may be because the asthma has entered a new phase; you should consult your doctor, who will modify the treatment. Or it may be that you have not managed to take the medicines on a regular basis, so that the delicate defences have been breached. The charts remind us how useful regular monitoring with a peak flow meter can be, so that a downward slide can be detected and reversed, for example with a short course of tablet steroids (Prednisolone). Chronic asthmatics are particularly exposed to the danger of the acute attack which can become dangerous if not checked, and a crisis plan is essential, worked out in advance with your doctor. Many people are worried about using steroids, and I have shown (on page 74) how the side effects can largely be avoided. Oral steroid tablets can be restricted to short sharp courses or taken on a day-on, day-off basis. These short courses can be started in advance of an expected challenge which is likely to be more severe than usual.

If a preventive shield of regular treatment with inhaled steroids is used, then this may be sufficient to prevent night asthma and early morning wheezes. If these persist, the doctor may consider prescribing slow-release tablets of theophylline (say, Nuelin, Slo-Phyllin or Theo-Dur) or salbutamol (Volmax or Spandets), taken before the night's rest. The aim will be to bring the night-time peak flow levels closer to the daytime levels; and after a time the extra treatment may become unnecessary.

It is all too easy to forget to take the medicine, especially in the middle of a busy working day. Four puffs of Becotide taken twice a day are as effective as two puffs taken four times a day; and one puff of Becloforte has five times the dosage of one puff of Becotide. If you leave your inhaler by your bedside or washstand, it will help you get into the habit of taking your night-time and early morning medication.

Cold air and exercise

The medicines need all the help they can get if they are to keep inflammation at bay. Background central heating is a necessity and, if not affordable all the time, can be switched on in the early morning and in the evening, with local heating for the rooms in use. An even temperature helps a great deal. A motor car often provides a convenient refuge when bringing an attack under control away from home. Shopping in winter is a special challenge; you can minimize the inherent problems by patronizing shops that are close at hand and by wearing a muffler. It can also be a good idea to avoid crowded places in the snuffly seasons.

Keeping fit is a real problem for the older chronic asthmatic. A leaflet published by the Chest, Heart and Stroke Association advises us to: 'Take a regular daily walk. Do not shuffle, a longer stride is more economical than a short one. Do not let your family fetch and carry for you, when you can do this job yourself. Do not take a lift if you can manage the stairs.' It is a good idea to take a couple of puffs of bronchodilator before setting out; if this does not work, then indoor exercise is recommended as an alternative: 'Choose where to exercise. This can be a staircase, or a passageway. Climb up and down the stairs or walk on the flat at a speed which makes you breathless, but not enough to make you stop.'

Physiotherapists are not too keen on generalized exercises, since people differ in their age, degree of fitness and the severity of their asthma. And it takes a very dedicated soul to exercise alone at home. Far better to join a class with others; but this also has its drawbacks, since the others may have normal airways and leave you far behind. To overcome this, one of the branches of the Asthma Society, at Twickenham, has set up classes in the multi-exercise gymnasium in the Adult Community College. The exercises have been devised with the help of a physiotherapist from the local hospital and are run by a P.E. teacher. Fifteen asthmatics attend, their ages ranging from the thirties to the seventies, and the emphasis is on individual programmes, carefully supervised, using weights from five kilos. There are many benefits, including improved peak flow readings and an ability to tolerate many more physical activities. It seems likely that this idea will soon spread to other areas.

Asthma related to work

It has long been known that certain occupations are associated with asthma; one of the earliest to be recognized was bakers' asthma, due to handling flour. 'Occupational asthma' in the strict sense is an illness which exists as a result of the work and is a 'prescribed' disease. Compensation for the ill-health can be obtained in the United Kingdom from the Department of Health and Social Security, provided:

- the substance complained of is listed for compensation

- the substance is present at work

- it can be shown by a doctor that your asthma has been caused by sensitivity to this agent

It can be difficult to detect work-related asthma if, as is often the case, the symptoms are experienced not at the workplace but in the evening or at night. One tell-tale sign is that symptoms fade away during the weekend or when on holiday, though it may take a few days for this to happen.

It is rare for the asthma to develop when you first come into contact with the offending substance. It may begin weeks, months or even years later. In some industries the asthma is allergic, and this can be demonstrated with a skin prick test. In others the mechanism is obscure. Generally speaking, asthma associated with animals or plants is allergic and asthma associated with chemicals is not. Occupational asthma can be aggravated by cigarette smoking.

The paint sprayer's tale

John Smith worked happily (we may suppose) as a paint sprayer for many years. He had no symptoms of wheeziness until, at the age of fifty, he was introduced to a new

paint system which used isocyanates as a hardener. There
were warnings on the can, but these were in German.
There was a ventilation system at work, but not a very
effective one, and when the wind blew from the east it
went into reverse.
John Smith became wheezy in the evenings but improved
at the weekends. A year later the asthma had become
severe. His G.P. referred him to a chest unit and a
'challenge test' using the suspected hardener confirmed
that it was to blame.
The prescription? Simply a change of job, though it took a
month for the symptoms to fade away.

It may sometimes be possible to replace the offending
substance with a safer material. If this is not possible, it may be
feasible to close off the equipment or to fit really effective fume-
extractors or to wear a mask.

Unfortunately, workers are often reluctant to cause a fuss,
and employers tend to become indignant if it is suggested that
their process is harmful. Tact is needed by the doctor who
investigates. On the other hand, a change of occupation usually
results in an end to the problem – unless the asthma is also caused
by other triggers encountered outside the workplace.

Claiming compensation

First consult your general practitioner. He may refer you to
hospital for special tests. If the doctors support the view that you
have occupational asthma, you then apply (in the United Kingdom)
to the Department of Health and Social Security (D.H.S.S.) for
Form NI. 237, which you return to them after you have filled it
in. If they decide you are eligible, they will ask you to attend for
examination by two doctors; eventually, if the D.H.S.S. supports
your claim, they will decide on the level of disablement. You may
appeal against their adverse decision to a tribunal.

The following list of eligible employments is not exhaustive
and is included to illustrate the kind of agents that may be
responsible for 'occupational asthma'.

Employment	Agent
the farming, milling and baking of grain/flour	grain or flour contaminated with grain weevils, mites or fungal spores
the milling and joinery of wood	wood dust (especially Western Red Cedar)
manufacture of 'biological' detergents and antibiotics	dust from enzymes and antibiotics
laboratory work with animals or insects	urine of rats, mice and guinea pigs; locusts
plastics, paints, adhesives and glues	various chemicals (isocyanates, formaldehyde, epoxy resins, acid anhydride)
refining metals	nickel, chromium, cobalt, platinum
electronics	colophony fumes from soldering fluxes
hairdressing	henna and bleaches

All the above are eligible for compensation if asthma results from exposure to the agent.

Chapter Seven

LIVING WITH FOOD ALLERGY

Is this a common cause of asthma?

At present it is widely believed that a whole range of illnesses can be ascribed to food allergy. As far as asthma is concerned, the verdict is a mixed one. The experts tell us that food is a much less common trigger for asthma than allergens (such as house dust mite) or irritants (such as infections). On the other hand, it was recently established at the Hammersmith Hospital in London that in children with a family history of asthma (especially among children of Indian parentage), the 'hyper-responsiveness' of their breathing tubes can be heightened by some foods in common use.

Food allergy can at times be an immediate and dramatic event. There may be a swelling of the lips and tongue, or an itchy rash, or headache, or pains in the stomach. More rarely, there can be coughing and wheezing. The remedy, where a single food is thought to be responsible, is simply to avoid that food in the future.

An allergic reaction to food may be delayed. This happens when it is caused, not by the food in its ingested state, but by the products which result when we digest it. This makes detection much more difficult.

The gut is where the allergic reaction to food starts. The offending food antigen is able to penetrate the thin skin (**epithelium**) and so enter the intestine and become absorbed in the bloodstream. The immune system recognizes the intruding antigen. In 'normal' people, no further action takes place. But in people who are 'atopic', there may be a vigorous response, even if the invader is no more harmful than the white of an egg. IgE antibodies are produced and attach to the local mast cells and basophils. These release various chemicals, such as histamine; among the many possible responses, a shortage of breath may occur due to a constriction of the breathing tubes.

Any naturally derived food can cause an allergic response, but it is the protein or carbohydrate component which provides the antigen. In children, the foods most commonly responsible are citrus fruits, apples, tomatoes, milk, white of egg, fish (especially shellfish), nuts (for example, peanut butter), chocolate, wheat products and yeasts (such as Marmite), peas, and many spices including ginger in biscuits. As the food-allergic child grows older, so the symptoms become less frequent, and most foods are well tolerated. The exceptions are egg white, fish and nuts, which may continue to produce reactions. Reactions to milk are mostly limited to early infancy.

Food intolerance caused by additives

Food may lead to asthmatic symptoms even when no allergic mechanism is involved; in this case there is a direct, irritating effect; for example, sodium metabisulphate is widely used as a preservative in soft drinks. As soon as the child takes a drink from the can or bottle there is a fit of coughing or wheeze. Mineral water does not produce this reaction.

The supermarket chains are well aware that many of their customers are concerned about food additives. Safeway Food Stores employ a Nutrition Advisory Service, and they have produced free booklets on additives. Booklet No.1 explains why they are used:

- to enable the food to be prepared more easily
- to make it taste or look better
- to prevent it from going stale
- to preserve the nourishment

It seems that the range of additives is vast. The booklet describes the role (among others) of antioxidants, preservatives, bulking agents, emulsifiers, crisping agents, stabilizers, thickening agents, sweeteners, flavours, colours and added nutrients. Many of these are both natural and harmless. Their second booklet explains what the EEC codes ('E' numbers) represent. It also puts a star against those additives which may, in sensitive individuals, cause adverse reactions such as asthma.

The food *colour* which is of greatest importance to asthmatics is the yellow Azo dye, tartrazine (E102). This turns up in syrups and soft drinks, in cakes, biscuits and puddings, in sauces and confectionery, in packet snacks, toppings and pickles. It is also used in medicines to make them yellow, green or orange.

The food *preservative* which causes most trouble in sensitive individuals is the one already mentioned: sodium metabisulphate (E223 and E224). This breaks down into the irritating gas, sulphur dioxide. It is not a natural substance, and it is used in acidic foods to prevent bacteria from growing, to preserve the colour and to maintain Vitamin C. Avoiding this colour is not easy, since it is added to beverages, dried fruits and vegetables, sausages, fresh prawns, fruit yoghurt, salad dressings, toppings, jams and flavouring essences.

Metabisulphate is also used in wines, along with salicylates, another trigger which affects some asthmatics. Wines are very complex drinks and contain many potentially allergenic substances, as well as the additives; for example, champagne contains yeasts which can upset some people. Pure alcohol is harmless but whisky and gin contain natural flavours that can cause wheeziness. Beers and ciders also contain preservatives, though in smaller amounts when they are canned. Some drinks, for example Coca Cola, can also cause asthma by virtue of the fact that they are acidic. So it may well be true, to adapt a famous quotation, that 'one man's drink is another man's poison'.

Equally difficult to pin down are the natural products which can cause asthma in infants, and which are used as carriers for flavourings. Examples include whey powder, dried skimmed milk and lactose. None of these has to be declared on the contents label.

Is salt to blame?

There is one additive that has been used since ancient times, at least among those tribes that abandoned the nomadic life and took up agriculture: salt. It has recently been suggested that there may be a link between a high intake of salt and a susceptibility to asthma. At a recent conference, Dr Peter Burney showed two maps of the English counties: the first was shaded to represent the local death-rate from asthma, and the second to show the average purchases of salt in all forms, including convenience foods which contain it. The two maps seemed to be almost identical. Both salt intake and the asthma death-rate were higher in the South-East and in the South. Could this be connected with the fact that in these areas there is a greater consumption of convenience foods? Here we are in the realms of conjecture, and more work will be needed before salt is either cleared of suspicion or finally incriminated. Low sodium salt is available at good health food shops.

Should asthmatics avoid certain foods?

This is a matter for debate among specialists. Patients' own reports of food intolerance have often been exaggerated. On the other hand, the interval between the meal and the appearance of the symptoms varies a good deal, so that genuine links reported by patients may be misbelieved. There are challenge tests, but these are suspect.

According to scientists reporting to the European Community, allergic reactions to foods such as milk, fish and nuts, affect between one-half and one per cent of the population, or about ten per cent of people who are atopic. They calculate that food additives affect only one-fifth of one per cent. About one child in 1,000 is sensitive to tartrazine and for most people, additives are harmless.

A diet based on fresh foods is a sensible alternative to one based on prepared foods, if these are suspected. And if in any case the patient's asthma is well controlled by the use of preventive medicines, then the wheeziness due to food or food additives is likely to be avoided at the same time.

Patients who react strongly to foods usually do so within a few minutes; if additives are suspected, the packet will list them (or most of them!) so that they can be identified. At Guy's Hospital in London, Professor Lessof has set up a National Data Bank which shows the components of the prepared foods in daily use, and your doctor can refer to this if in doubt.

Are there any reliable tests?

For the most part, allergists rely not on tests but on case-histories. These require persistence and skill because asthmatics tend to forget their occasional lapses (when the forbidden food was eaten) and they tend to respond too readily to prompts by the investigator. Careful probing is needed to arrive at the truth.

Laboratory tests are mainly used to confirm the findings of case-histories and, if positive, to convince all concerned that the suspect food was indeed responsible for the asthma. Generally speaking, these tests are not helpful, either because the materials do not reproduce the food accurately or because the reaction was due to breakdown products. It is therefore wise to be sceptical about laboratory tests which are advertised commercially.

The allergist has to be careful to eliminate other possible triggers: the food may appear only in a certain house where there are also animals which are not encountered at home.

Are elimination diets helpful?

In the days before modern medicines were introduced, complicated elimination diets were recommended by physicians. There are various ways in which these can be carried out. One is to start with a diet of foods which seldom cause allergy. If the symptoms improve, other foods are introduced in stages until the offending food is discovered. There are some objections to this procedure:

• The diets bring only temporary relief because they do not eliminate the underlying tendency to have asthma.

• If the diet is continued for a long period, the patient may suffer from a lack of essential nutrients. In children this may restrict growth; for example, there may be a loss of zinc and calcium, of total proteins, and of Vitamin D.

• People with food allergy are usually allergic to inhaled allergens as well, and the medicines used to control these reactions are likely to control the food allergy at the same time.

However, there is one kind of food allergy in which a restricted 'exclusion' diet may be justified. This is where the connection with a particular food is not obvious and the asthma is severe. The diet must be carried out under medical supervision. And the diagnosis is confirmed by giving the suspected food in a disguised form and then carrying out breathing tests for a few days. If the exclusion diet produces no response in a couple of weeks it is abandoned.

Is breast feeding desirable?

The latest evidence suggests that mother's milk does give some protection against the development of an atopic illness and, surprisingly, diminishes any extra risk which might otherwise arise from the mother herself being atopic. The small amounts of antigen present in formulas based on cow's milk can provoke an allergic response. Breast feeding can also reduce the risk of virus infections. For the first three months, the mother's consumption of cow's milk should be reduced but not eliminated, because that would deprive mother and child of essential calcium. In these early days the mother should also avoid the kind of foods that can cause reactions: fish, nuts and cereals, especially if either or both parents are atopic. Switching to soy milk will make no difference in preventing asthma or other atopic disorders such as eczema; goat's milk is not suitable for young babies and casein hydrolysate, which is derived from cow's milk, is suitable – but at the same time foul-tasting and expensive.

Dieting during pregnancy (for example, in a second pregnancy when the first child has developed asthma) is not only unnecessary but also is to be discouraged, since the mother needs all the nutrients that are available in a balanced diet when she is pregnant.

Overweight asthmatics

Asthmatics notice that their wheeziness gets worse after a heavy meal; this is because a distended stomach presses on the diaphragm. There is another reason for avoiding large meals, if these result in becoming overweight. This extra weight has to be carried around and this needs extra energy, which the lungs have to provide by supplying extra oxygen. In asthma this supply is limited, so the overweight asthmatic will be at a greater disadvantage than the asthmatic who keeps slim, with or without exercise.

Conclusion

There are various ways in which asthma caused by diet can be reduced or eliminated:

- by identifying and avoiding the offending substance
- by trying out an 'exclusion' diet under strict medical supervison
- by the regular use of preventive medicines taken for asthma due to all manner of triggers, of which food is only one
- breast feeding in infancy
- avoiding being overweight

As in all asthma treatments, the key to success is trial and observation under the supervision of your doctor.

Chapter Eight

LIVING WITH HAY FEVER

A common illness

As we have seen, the nose is a most efficient dust extractor. It removes most of the unwanted particles that enter, and it does so by creating a turbulence caused by its narrow entrance. This throws the air we breathe against a mucus blanket which lines the cavities and traps the particles. The nose also provides the correct temperature and amount of moisture for the air before it enters the lungs.

About one person in ten complains to the doctor that this mechanism has over-reacted. He or she is told that they have 'rhinitis', which simply means any persistent discharge from the nose. If watery and runny, it is known as 'rhinorrhoea'; if thick and congested, it is referred to as 'catarrh'. 'Hay fever' is the most frequently experienced form of rhinitis, and is both seasonal and due to allergy.

Some patients have rhinitis all the year round ('perennial rhinitis'). This may, like hay fever, be allergic in the strict sense that the triggers also show up on skin prick tests. If one or more of these is positive (for example, to house dust mite) you are said to be 'atopic'. On the other hand the discharge may be caused by irritants which do not show up on the skin tests, in which case you have 'non-atopic rhinitis'. Anyone who gets frequent head 'colds' in winter should ask the doctor whether these should be regarded as rhinitis, and treated as such.

In the ten-year period to 1981, consultations for rhinitis and for asthma doubled, which suggests that airborne pollutants have increased. Among boys rhinitis is most common when they are aged between five and fifteen. Among girls, it is the fifteen-to-twenty age-group that suffers most. Rhinitis is particularly common among asthmatics; in half the sufferers, it disappears – and, for some obscure reason, this often follows a particularly bad year. In most cases it lessens as we grow older and our immune responses become weaker.

What does it feel like?

The symptoms range from a few itchy sneezes while walking to work to something very like a fever, though the temperature stays normal. It is like having a head cold in its most distressing phase, with the added torment of intense irritation, as if a thousand tiny needles were at work in your eyes and nose. You feel as if your head is about to explode. There are fever-like shivers. Your handkerchief quickly soaks and your nose becomes red and sore. The constant sneezing is embarrassing. In addition, there is a feeling of unease and tiredness. Inflammation in the nasal passages can lead to blocked sinuses and, if these become infected, you may lose your sense of smell and have severe pains in the face. In childhood it is especially unfortunate that hay fever reaches a peak during the June examinations, diminishing both concentration and self-confidence. When you have hay fever, you want to be left alone, whether child or adult.

In more clinical terms these symptoms can be summarized as:

• in the nose: 'rhinitis'. A copious discharge of runny or congested mucus; sneezing, soreness and inflammation. Pain in the face shows that the sinuses are blocked. There may be headaches.

• in the eyes: 'conjunctivitis'. They become itchy, red and swollen.

• in the throat: 'pharyngitis'. This too is itchy and sore and, at the height of the pollen season, there is a tendency to cough and wheeze.

In my recollection of childhood, hay fever and asthma were never equally severe on the same day. Sunny weather seemed to release the pollens and brought on the hay fever. Damp, rainy weather washed away the pollen, but switched on the asthma instead. Perhaps this had been triggered by the previous day's hay fever, or there may have been a greater release of mould spores on the damp days.

What are the triggers?

The triggers for 'hay fever' are of course seasonal, but rhinitis can occur all the year round. In Scotland, pollens are released a few weeks later than in England.

The seasonal triggers are:

• pollens from trees (especially plane and birch trees in April and May)

• pollens from grasses (especially timothy, rye and meadow grass from the end of May to the end of July)

• pollens from weeds (especially nettles and docks in July and August)

• pollens from flowers and shrubs (according to the flowering season)

• mould spores (released by fungi from grass mowings, in woods and forests and in old damp houses and furniture (from July to October)

If your symptoms start in February and March, you are probably allergic to pollens from trees. If you have allergic rhinitis in the autumn, then moulds should be suspected. Ornamental flowers in the garden are pollinated mainly by insects and their heavier pollen grains do not travel very far, though they can be a problem when brought into the house and placed by the bedside. The grasses, on the other hand, produce pollen which is wind-pollinated and can be carried for hundreds of miles, descending at last on cities as well as on farmland.

All year-round triggers include the ones already described in Chapter Two with suggestions as to how they may be avoided; house dust mite (especially from late autumn) and horses and furry pets. (Food allergy is not thought to be a common cause of allergic rhinitis.)

Non-allergic rhinitis can also occur all the year round, and the triggers include:

• air pollution (exhaust fumes, cigarette smoke, perfumes, sulphur dioxide from the burning of fossil fuels, smoke from a wood fire or frying food)

• the nose may run more when you take a hot drink or soup, and alcohol increases the flow of blood through the nose and makes it feel stuffy

• climate and temperature play a part, but this varies from one person to another. Extremes should be avoided: both the very dry air caused by central heating set at too high a level and a very humid climate

• women with rhinitis tend to feel worse when they are pregnant or taking oral contraceptives

• salicylates (not only in aspirin but also present in cheap wines) can cause rhinitis.

Why do some people suffer from allergic rhinitis?

The short answer is that they are over-sensitive to triggers such as pollens, in their nasal passages. There are two distinct stages; to be successful, preventive treatment should precede the first stage.

STAGE ONE: Pollen is trapped in the mucus lining of the nose. The chemicals from the pollen manage to penetrate the lining and reach white blood cells (lymphocytes) which circulate in the blood stream. These lymphocytes respond by producing IgE antibodies in large numbers. In time, these manage to attach themselves to mast cells, and by so doing form 'receptors' so that the mast cells are primed and ready for the next stage, like a pistol waiting to be discharged. At the same time, these mast cells manage to escape through the thin skin (epithelium) which lines the airways.

STAGE TWO: More pollen arrives, perhaps a few weeks later, and cross-links those IgE receptors in the manner described in Chapter One on page 22. This causes an explosion of the mast cells, so that they shoot out chemicals such as histamine in great quantities. These chemicals produce the symptoms of hay fever already described.

It seems that in 'normal' people the immune mechanism identifies the particles we breathe by means of 'T-cells'. If the particles are harmful, for example germs and viruses, they encourage the lymphocytes to form all those IgE antibodies. If on the other hand the intruders are quite harmless, like pollen grains and house dust particles, then the T-cells act instead as suppressors and no IgE antibodies are formed. It has been suggested that in allergic (atopic) individuals, the T-cells can promote the production of IgE but have no power to suppress it; so IgE is made inappropriately in response to pollen grains, possibly through a genetic defect.

It is also possible that virus infections, so common in early childhood, contribute to this malfunction. Once the level of IgE antibody circulating everywhere goes up, it remains at a high level and the mast cells are primed to respond to the next invasion of pollen grains and other atopic triggers.

Dr Robert Davies of St Bartholomew's Hospital, London, has described the fruits of recent research. Medical students who were atopic allowed tiny extracts to be taken from the tissues of their nostrils after pollen had been sprayed up them. The tissue extracts are stained so as to allow examination under the powerful electron microscope. This procedure is repeated at intervals.

This research has shown that as the hay fever season advances the mast cells increase eightfold and the proportion of mast cells which rise to the inner surface increases fourfold. This means that early in the pollen season the mast cells increase thirty-two times at the sites where they can respond most readily to the invading allergens.

Implications for treatment

This research, partly funded by the Asthma Research Council, has three important implications for sufferers:

• When trying to block the mast cells with medical treatment, do not wait until the peak pollen season in June but start in mid-May. Most sufferers first notice symptoms when the official pollen count rises to 'low'. They should delay no longer. If the spring is cooler or drier than usual, the pollen season will be earlier. If you are sensitive to tree pollens, you have to start as early as April.

• The main purpose of treatment will be to reduce inflammation in the air passages, and for this purpose the preferred method will be to use corticosteroids.

• If you manage to block one allergen (say, pollen) you will stand a good chance of blocking all the others (dust, moulds, dander) and there will be less of a risk that the rhinitis will continue into the autumn and winter.

The pollen count

In the United Kingdom this is measured on the roof of St Mary's Hospital, Paddington. It arrives, rather crudely, at the number of pollen grains in a cubic metre of air: 200 is regarded as 'high' and 50 as 'low'. The highest count ever in central London was 870, recorded on 17 June 1964. Hay fever sufferers are sensitive to quite low counts, especially when 'primed', and should rely on their own judgement as to how they will respond, assisted by the weather forecast.

The volume of pollens is affected by temperatures in the preceding winter and spring, because these govern the flowering of the plants. As far as any individual is concerned, it is also affected by the following factors: the direction of the prevailing wind; where you live; the extent to which you can exclude the pollens by closing the windows. The pollen count is highest in the early morning and in the late afternoon. This is because the pollen cloud lifts high into the air in the warm up-currents and descends again at night; so, if windows are to be opened, this should be done in the middle of the day.

Managing hay fever successfully

Can you take avoiding action? The answer is an emphatic 'YES'. There are three kinds of preventive measures.

• Take preventive medicines every day; and you should *start before the pollen season begins* and continue until it ends.

• Stay indoors as much as possible and keep the rooms cool and shaded and the windows shut, especially when the grass is being mown. Mowing the lawn releases millions of mould spores and should be left to someone else to do. (Paving stones might be a sensible long-term alternative.) Wear dark glasses to protect the eyes against dust as well as sunshine. Avoid cigarette smoke. If you are studying or sitting examinations, sit as far as possible from open windows.

• When choosing a holiday it seems best to go away at the height of the local pollen season if you can. At the seaside, the sea-breezes blow into the land and keep the pollens at bay. In mountainous country, the rising air-currents sweep up the sloping pastures and take the pollens with them. In Scandinavia the grass pollen counts are usually low, but avoid the May flowering of the forests of birch trees. House dust mites do not thrive in the dry air of the Alps, so skiers and walkers can enjoy a temporary respite from rhinitis.

Preventing the symptoms with medicines

A THE NOSE: (Before using a nasal spray, it is a good idea to clear the nose of the accumulated secretions.)

In order to prevent the mast cells from escaping and multiplying at the beginning of the season, start taking an aerosol spray delivering steroid when they are still in their winter quarters. Start in May and use night and morning. Continue until the end of the grass and weed pollen season, even when you have no symptoms. If you adopt this treatment it is highly unlikely that any symptoms will develop. (The brand names are: Beconase; Rynacort; Syntaris.) Another way of stabilizing the mast cells is to use Rynacrom (sodium chromoglycate) four times a day. This is more effective in young people and is used to supplement the steroids if these would otherwise have to be used in a higher dosage.

If the nose is blocked, use nasal steroid drops. These must be dropped into the nose with your head on the floor or hanging over the edge of a bed; the head should be kept *vertical* during this procedure. (Brand name: Becasol Nasal Drops.) These should also be taken every day.

You may start this treatment too late, when your nose is already blocked. Or you may find that the rhinitis persists into the autumn and winter. In this case you need a short course of tablet steroid, i.e. Prednisolone. Take 15 mg a day (three 5 mg tablets) for two weeks, and then stabilize on 5 mg a day plus the aerosol steroid. This technique is also useful if you want to keep your head clear for a special purpose such as taking examinations. Start two days before.

B THE EYES
(The eyes have to be treated separately from the nose.)

These can be treated with eye-drops. Opticrom stabilizes the mast cells and is very safe. But it has to be used four times a day for both seasonal and year-round rhinitis.

The preferred treatment nowadays is to use one of the newer anti-histamines such as Hismanal and Triludan. These can last for two or three days and produce very little drowsiness.

Tablet steroid (Prednisolone) will also reduce itchiness in the eyes, because the same mechanism is at work as in the nasal passages. Injections of cortisone (Depo-Medrone or Kenalog) are also used, since they last for up to six weeks. No other treatment is needed and this can tide you over the period of exams.

An eye-wash should be used before you take the Opticrom, to remove dirt and irritants.

Desensitization can be carried out by injecting pollen extracts given before the season starts and continued each season for two or three years. In non-seasonal rhinitis, dust mite extracts are used. The dangers of desensitization injections are discussed in Chapter Two on page 41. There is a risk of a severe reaction to the injections, and they tend be used only when the symptoms are (a) atopic; (b) really disabling; and (c) have not responded to other treatments.

Nasal polyp

This is a pale-grey structure which arises in the sinuses, then extends into the nose and causes a blockage. The polyp is caused when the nasal lining becomes swollen and attracts water, which leaks from the blood channels, and then proteins, which stretch the lining until it forms the polyp or sac. When the tissue recovers, the polyps can become blocked, and as a result the sinuses may also be infected. This can be acute, with pains in the head, or it may be longer-lasting, with a persistent drip of mucus into the nose. It can cause bad breath where there is an infection. As with nasal polyps, the treatment for the sinuses consists of dealing with the perennial rhinitis, using the medicines that have been described, with the possible addition of an antibiotic.

Snoring is another consequence of a stuffed-up nose, so a course of Beconase could be tried if this creates a social problem!

Unsuitable and unusual remedies

In 1881, 'Cigars of Joy' provided soothing substances. In 1891, hay fever could positively be cured by the Carbolic Smoke Ball! In 1936, a means was devised of passing radio waves through the head and I recall sitting between two glass spheres and listening to the whirring of the motor like the sound of a melancholy windscreen wiper. In the 1950s, people went on sea-cruises or took up hypnosis or installed air-purifiers. In the 1960s, a school was built underground in the U.S.A.

Decongestant drops are widely used to treat rhinitis – they should be avoided. They are designed to shrink the inflamed nasal lining and do so effectively, so that you feel better. Then there is a rebound and the inflammation returns, this time in a more severe form. So you take more drops. You end either by being permanently bunged up or the mucus blanket dries and leaves the linings exposed to germs. You pass from an acute phase into a more or less permanent condition, and this is unnecessary because there are excellent remedies, as have been described.

In the early 1980s there was a great deal of publicity for 'Bubbleheads'. These rest on the shoulders and allow the head to move freely inside. They are designed to protect asbestos workers and are provided with a filter which can remove pollen, dust and cigarette smoke down to half a micron. The inventor, who suffers from severe hay fever, claims that if the bubble is worn for 30–45 minutes in the morning (for example, when driving to work) and again in the evening, this will allow the nasal passages to recover so that they are much less sensitive at times when the bubble is not worn. At the time of writing, the price of the Bubblehead is £180 and the address can be found at the back of the book under 'Useful Addresses'.

Chapter Nine

THE HUMAN RESPONSE

As seen by others

Perhaps the most distressing aspect of asthma and hay fever when not well controlled is the way they can mess up normal human relationships, the ones everyone else takes for granted. The sufferers appear to be fit and well, yet even when the symptoms are mild they can behave at times as if they are invalids. They reasonably decline to take part in activities which to the non-asthmatic seem to present no kind of threat. Children, in particular, are under suspicion that they sometimes use their illness to obtain favours or to avoid unpleasant tasks; but this may in fact be a reasonable defence against challenges which have, in the past, shown them up as inadequate. This is especially so in a society which applauds achievements in sports and games above all else.

The way each of us sees our own illness is, whether we like it or not, powerfully affected by the way other people see it. Asthmatics are often astonished at the response which casual acquaintances make when the illness is mentioned: the asthmatic is informed, with an air of authority, that the illness 'is all due to nerves'. For some reason, hay fever is ascribed not to nerves but to pollens, though the mechanisms are similar! On the other hand, the response may go to the opposite extreme and suggest a crippling disease which is a kind of life-sentence.

To obtain a detached view of these attitudes, I persuaded a friend who carries out 'group discussions' for commercial purposes to conclude a few sessions with the topic, 'How do you view asthma as an illness?' There were separate groups for adults and for children, and no asthmatics were present. The views expressed are given here as direct quotations.

Adult manual workers tended to be both realistic and fatalistic:

• 'An asthmatic's lung capacity is a lot lower than a normal person's.'

• 'I have a cousin who was pensioned off at 22 because of asthma.'

• 'My step-brother lost his job as a park keeper, just couldn't breathe.'

• 'Most people rate it at three [on a scale of ten] but I rate it at nine.'

White-collar respondents on the other hand came across as rather dismissive:

• 'One of my son's friends gets it, so as soon as he walks through the door we say "Have you got your inhaler?" Really it's up to the individual to control it.'

• 'I've seen kids running around and getting short of breath, but one little squirt and they're as right as rain. I'd have thought in ninety-nine per cent of cases it is only an inconvenience.'

• 'The people I've known with asthma, one puff and they're O.K.'

The children were either completely unaware ('Is it the same as hay fever? . . . as eczema?') or concerned and observant:

• 'I used to baby-sit for a child with asthma and it was awful – you think they are going to die in front of you.'

• 'He's like an animal on the football field but all the precautions he takes before, blowing his nose, puffing away, you'd think he wasn't going to last six months.'

• 'They hate people fussing – all those people round her and you could see she wanted them to go away.'

• 'This girl at school almost goes blue because she doesn't want to use the inhaler, so we all shout at her when we see her go like that.'

It is in the schools where the biggest advances in understanding can be made.

Asthma as seen by parents

The general lack of understanding as to the true nature of asthma bears especially heavily on parents of asthmatic children; I asked two friends with experience of asthma in very young children to describe their worries and frustrations.

The only two people I had known who had asthma had died from it, so when I was told my baby might be asthmatic I was quite frankly terrified. I did not know where to turn for informed advice. The most that family and friends could offer was a few words of 'Poor you' and 'Oh dear!' and they simply did not want to become involved. Asthma is not nice to talk about, unless there are several asthmatics in the family, and then you get the old wives' tales and the attitude: 'You've just got to put up with it, my dear . . . nothing can be done about it.' It can take a parent a long time to learn how to cope with an asthmatic child. Each parent needs the other's support; it must be very hard indeed for one parent if the other is unsympathetic or simply does not want to know: unfortunately, not an uncommon experience. I know of marriages that have failed because of the strain of coping with asthma.

The second mother's account also stresses the sense of isolation, but this can bring a strengthening of the marriage:

If they have an asthmatic child, parents have to cope with a feeling of failure. There is the nagging thought that 'if only that chest infection had been cleared up asthma would never have developed'. Added to that there is a sort of character assassination by friends who hint that the child is over-indulged and playing up, using the illness to obtain sympathy, a 'typical asthmatic'. In reality there are nerve-racking moments, as when you have to administer a nebulizer and the child is terrified of the noise it makes. Problems with diets (no eggs) means turning up at all the children's parties and this receives adverse comment. Then you have to worry about the non-asthmatic sister or brother who has to compete for the mother's attention and does so by being aggressive. The sad thing is that you can lose a lot of friends through having an asthmatic child . . . but this does bring the family very close together.

Another mother has written: 'When a severe attack occurs I

have to go into automatic control in order to be able to cope, and this is followed by complete exhaustion, physically and emotionally, while the child has become quite relaxed and active.'

It is an understatement to say that asthma has its ups and downs. Parents take a year or two to learn how to manage their child's asthma. Everything seems to be well controlled – then, out of the blue, the child has a sudden severe attack for which there seems to be no clear explanation. This is deeply unsettling. The parents feel that they must start all over again, learning how to manage the asthma. As one mother has put it, 'The first dash to Casualty after a long period of relative calm can reduce the parents to the same nervous, unsure, guilty state they were in when the asthma was first diagnosed.'

From the child's viewpoint

In my childhood, asthma was thought not to be preventable and, like tuberculosis, to require copious draughts of fresh air, by day and by night. At school, conformity was all-important, and in those days success at games was essential for self-esteem. Failure to shine on windy playing fields tended to make one an 'outsider', and it is hard for children to be cast aside because of their essential nature.

Nowadays preventive medicine can allow play to be both normal and natural. Children with asthma can learn to tolerate exercise of increasing severity, provided the steps towards this are gradual. If barred from games, a child may lose a great deal. As Freud wrote; 'Our sense of identity is rooted in our physical being.' Play is essential for the development of all young primates, whether apes or gorillas, or human children. Play stimulates, enables children to feel that they belong and develops social skills. It provides opportunities for laughter and tears, teaches endurance and tests aspects of personality.

Over- and under-protection

At a meeting of a self-help group, there was sympathy for the mother who, though aware of the dangers of being either too hard or too soft on her asthmatic daughter, admitted that she tended to swing from one extreme to the other and back again. Keeping an even balance between the two is not at all easy.

Parents sometimes feel that their children are only pretending to wheeze, in order to gain attention. But the pretend wheeze can physiologically trigger a real attack. A child may 'forget' to use the inhaler, and this produces a genuine wheeze, which gives the same result. It is therefore possible for some families to become caught up in a cycle from which neither parents nor child can escape. This is why a stay in hospital or with relatives can by itself make a child's asthma better. A parent has written:

> It is very natural to panic when you see your child struggle for breath ... No doubt you will resolve to fight against another attack, even another attack occurring. But isolating your child from infection, not allowing the child to take part in strenuous exercise, and not applying discipline lest the emotional upset brings on an attack, is not going to help. The child needs to know that he is as good as his peers, and should not regard himself as 'delicate'.

Parents with an asthmatic child who is strong-willed and assertive face a special kind of challenge, one that has been described by a mother in these words:

> Since our third child developed asthma some years ago, as a three-year-old, our family has lurched from crisis to crisis. I was terrified that he would die, because the attacks were dangerously severe, and he has become the centre of our life. After many months his condition was brought under control, although he was ill more often than not. He has a will of iron. No doubt we spoiled him, and family life centred around his needs. As he grew older he became a tyrant, an expert manipulator, insisting on playing football on damp days when it made him ill, and the illness then demanded total attention. My two older children became second-class citizens in our home, selflessly protecting their demanding younger brother.

> Finally, I arranged to visit a psychiatrist. He did not blame me but pointed out that, in spite of the attention, our son has felt different and therefore isolated from the rest of the family. We should in future treat him as any other child, showing no more interest in his asthma attacks than we would a cold or sore throat in the other children. If he behaves like a two-year-old he should be treated the way a two-year-old is treated. There would be no more get-well presents ...

Things are much better now; he is taking different drugs and his asthma is more controlled, itself a factor in the improvement in his behaviour.

From the adolescent's viewpoint

Adolescence is a difficult time, even without a disability such as asthma. It is a time when self-confidence is put to the test; additionally there are hormonal changes which, in girls, bring with them a monthly cycle, and this can itself influence the ups and downs of asthma.

Teenagers want, above all, to be like – and to be liked by – their companions. They want to be able to join in everything, including games, dances and crowded parties. Any one of these can bring on wheeziness, for example just rushing out into the cold from a disco dance. Teenagers are reluctant to be seen using their inhalers, so may neglect to do so. As Gerald Scarfe, the cartoonist, severely asthmatic in childhood, mentioned in his autobiographical film: 'I was ashamed of my illness, because it made me feel different.' At times the asthmatic teenager has to stand and watch while others play.

Teenagers attach more importance to good company than to good health. It is as hard to persuade them to give up smoking as to take the medicines prescribed. They do not want to be reminded of these restrictions at a time when their peers are demonstrating what Professor Milner aptly calls 'fatalistic bravado'.

What role can the parents play? Their advice on any topic is unwelcome; it is felt by their teenage children that parents cannot possibly understand the emotional upsets and upheavals. I asked a mother who is at present coping with a teenage asthmatic to provide an answer. She has written:

> I think it is important to see the problem as a whole, and not just from the viewpoint of asthma. When children reach their eleventh or twelfth year we parents should take time to talk to them about the difficulties they will face, explain that they will reject parental advice on many matters and that they will have to be strong and rely on their own code of self-discipline.

Let them begin to manage their own asthma at an early age: ten years old is not too young. Teach them how to use a peak flow meter, how to check whether their inhaler is full or nearly empty, and that they know when to use it. Try to make them understand that asthma is a common illness which they have to accept and learn how to control by themselves so that for most of the time the disadvantages become quite bearable.

Are there any suitable films, videos or audio tapes? Fisons have produced videos with the titles: 'A Breath of Fresh Air', 'Asthma in the Family' and 'Why Do I Wheeze?', and Allen & Hanbury offer 'Understanding Asthma' and 'Every Little Breath'. All these are on VHS video tape and can be borrowed from a local branch of the Asthma Society by a member.

There is one aspect of education which may become neglected in the teenage years, in all children, not merely by asthmatics. It is surely unfortunate that the creative abilities, carefully fostered in the primary schools, tend to wither away during adolescence, especially when schools are deprived of funds to devote to the arts. In later life I have derived great consolation from creative pursuits begun in my teens. I talked about this to an asthma group in Chelmsford and a member of the audience agreed emphatically: 'When I am painting I forget about asthma completely.' Crafts taken up in childhood and skills acquired in the teenage years can provide an absorbing interest for a lifetime. As Sir Winston Churchill wrote: 'Painting is a friend who makes no undue demands, excites to no exhausting pursuits, keeps faithful pace even with feeble steps.'

As seen by adults

Asthma can start or reappear at any age; when first made, the diagnosis can be as unsettling at fifty as at an earlier age. There is no chance of 'growing out' of late onset asthma, and it appears to the sufferer to be a kind of life sentence. It is all too easy to adopt a fatalistic approach and to give in too easily, especially if, in the early stages, the treatments are not successful.

If it is any consolation, my own asthma went out of control in my mid-fifties. What should I do? Should I give up my job or move to a warmer climate? In the event I pestered the doctors to teach me how the medicines were supposed to work. After three years of trial and error I learned how to use them effectively and also how to avoid a wide range of triggers. As a result, I can now move around, continue to earn a living and draw comfort from the fact that those very severe attacks are now less frequent.

Relatively little has been written by asthmatics about their own illness. Dr Anthony Storr, in his illuminating foreword to *Asthma The Facts*, gives a convincing and moving account of what it is like to experience severe asthma, his dislike of having to take the medicines each day and the adjustments that have to be made.

As seen by psychiatrists

Is there an 'asthmatic personality'?

It would not be surprising if asthmatics – at least those with a severe form of the illness – were to develop some neurotic traits and acquire a reputation for being eccentric. But it seems that, by and large, asthmatics are neither more nor less neurotic than the population at large.

In 1970, Dr Andrew Zealley and colleagues in Edinburgh examined the personalities of three groups of people, using standard tests to discover neurotic tendencies. One group was super-normal (they had no neurotic traits); a second group was drawn from people known to be neurotic; the third was composed of seventy asthmatics, selected on a random basis. The asthmatic group emerged as being neither more nor less obsessional, over-sensitive and over-anxious than normal people; in other words, they were mid-way between the two control groups; they were much less neurotic than the neurotic group. Only in one category was their score higher than 'normal': they tended to lack self-confidence. It is hardly a matter for wonder that an illness which strikes at the air supply, at the basis of life itself, and does so for days on end, should diminish self-confidence.

There is one way in which asthma can interfere directly

with ordinary relationships. Some asthmatics, from childhood onwards, tend to talk rapidly and to pause in mid sentence. If a friend tries to fill in this gap, the asthmatic either subsides completely or overrides the interruption as soon as the missing breath arrives, appearing to be over-assertive but in reality feeling at a disadvantage.

Can psychotherapy help?

Asthma may be triggered by stress and may itself be a source of profound anxiety. Any doctor who takes the trouble to listen to an asthmatic patient's problems and explain how the illness can be controlled will do much to allay the anxiety. As we shall see, there are sensible ways of relieving stress and dealing with everyday problems.

Psychotherapy in its strict sense can be used to relieve asthma in two kinds of situation. The first is where the asthma is reinforced by a profound, perhaps buried anxiety which, if identified and faced, will disappear and so remove a cause of the asthma. The second is where a patient, perhaps unconsciously, is using the asthma to manipulate another member of the family. If this is brought into the open and recognized, then the symptoms may diminish. Depressive illnesses are treated not with psychotherapy but with the appropriate drugs.

Is asthma in any sense 'psychosomatic'?

Translated into plain English, this question is really asking whether the top brain can directly influence the workings of the lungs. There is plenty of evidence from the medical literature that it can do so, by a conditioned response. A very suggestible asthmatic may become wheezy when presented with, say, a perfectly formed artificial rose or a picture of a cat – if the equivalent real objects produce this response. Relief from an inhaler may be afforded in some patients, even when an inert substance has been substituted for the active drug. Quite recently at St Thomas's hospital in London it was shown that a film depicting horrifying scenes caused reduced peak flow in the asthmatic patients who saw it. All this does support the view that the top brain is 'wired up' to the nerves which cause spasm in the bronchial tubes. But these responses can take place only if the subject is asthmatic in the first place; this does not prove that asthma is a 'nervous condition'. There are many other triggers which may cause wheeziness, and it is only a minority of asthmatics who react to 'dummy' allergens.

Suffering in silence

A doctor in general practice and trained in psychiatry, after surveying his own patients and those in neighbouring practices, has reported that asthmatics, far from using their illness to demand attention when it is not needed, are generally reluctant to seek help when they should do so. They prefer to manage by themselves. This has led some psychoanalysts to suppose that asthma develops out of conflicts which arose in childhood and are then bottled up, especially conflicts with demanding parents. However, as Dr Storr has pointed out, these conflicts are experienced by all children, so they cannot be responsible for asthma, which is suffered by only a few.

Most physical conditions are influenced by stress: headaches are one obvious example, and we can become breathless with excitement. The kind of stress that can contribute to asthma is, according to trained observers, seldom the short sharp stress but is more likely to be the long-drawn-out family row, or continuing worry about exams, or mounting pressures and rising fatigue at work. People vary a great deal in the amount of stress they can handle, and asthmatics vary a good deal in their perception as to how severe their own symptoms are. One is totally disrupted by only mild asthma while another leads a normal life, even though afflicted by asthma which is at times severe.

Four ways of relieving stress

In older children, resentment arising from asthma is likely to be expressed not in words but in aggressive behaviour, such as the slamming of a door in response to a quite reasonable request.

This is perfectly natural, and there is no way parents can or should try to prevent their children from getting upset. No one can protect a child (or an adult) from the normal reactions to stress: anger, worry and excitement. Instead:

• Encourage the child (or adult) to talk about the stress or worry and quite literally 'get it off his chest'. This may require the subtle tactic of referring to your own frustration and asking whether the feelings are shared.

• If there are family quarrels, try to sort the out – with outside help if need be.

• Encourage the asthmatic to find out which physical stresses can and which cannot be tolerated. When choosing a recreation, sport or career, aim to avoid as many of the stressful situations as possible.

• Encourage relaxation techniques of any kind. When we are tense, the muscles get tense – including the bronchial muscles. The exercises can be practised from the age of five upwards and should be made enjoyable. As has already been mentioned, swimming is particularly good for asthmatics: it requires controlled breathing, it helps people to relax and 'let off steam', and promotes self-confidence.

A mother has written: 'Parents who do not talk to their children about asthma are doing the child a disservice. Even quite young children with the illness can be reassured if the treatment is explained in simple terms. At the same time, be calm and positive about the illness. Do not allow the child's asthma to take over or transmit any of your worries [about the asthma] to the child.'

Making friends with the health professionals

The general practitioner's role

It is natural, given their sense of isolation and sometimes of despair, that asthmatics and parents should seek from their doctors the kind of support that may be lacking elsewhere. It is, however, rare for doctors to be trained in this kind of counselling; they concentrate on physical causes and medicines and tend not to want to become involved with all the factors that may contribute to the illness in the home.

Attitudes are changing. Practitioners are beginning to teach asthmatic patients preventive medicine, how to use the equipment and to monitor the result with a peak flow meter. They are beginning to supply crisis management cards which show how the treatment should be adapted to meet a deterioration, and to insist on recall visits to the surgery, whether or not the symptoms are well controlled. Practice nurses – and indeed nurses generally – are being trained to listen to patients' problems so that the patterns of asthma can be better understood and challenged. Simply to have a sympathetic listener can sow the seed of confidence. An advance on these fronts is likely to bring the biggest improvements in the management of asthma in the next decade or two, rather than the development of radically new medicines.

Make a friend of your doctor. Try to save his time by jotting down beforehand the questions you want to ask. If they are numerous, ask for an extended consulting time. The doctor cannot teach you all he knows, nor even a part of it – and in any case he has to cover a huge range of illnesses, many of them as complicated as asthma. It is up to you to find out as much as you can if the treatments are not working.

If you cannot obtain the answers you need either from books and leaflets or from the brief consultations with your own doctor, then you should ask for a referral to the hospital. You may also change your doctor; a list can be obtained from the local Family Practitioner's Committee, and your chemist will have their address.

The local pharmacist

People who are worried about their medicines often fail to realize that their local pharmacist or dispensing chemist is not only well versed in the possible side effects but is very willing to explain what these are, the purpose of the medicines and the correct way to take them. Asthma drugs are among those most commonly prescribed, and pharmacists can attend refresher courses on the treatment of asthma.

In time of need

There are various ways in which people with chronic severe asthma, or those looking after them, may be able to alleviate real financial hardship caused by the illness. These are liable to change; on 11 April 1988 Supplementary Benefit was replaced by Income Support. This eliminated some of the extra payments for which asthma sufferers might be eligible and for single payments substituted the Budget Fund which, for example, provides loans to enable people to buy equipment.

If you need information about any of the D.H.S.S. benefits, write to your local office. Local Authority social workers will be able to tell you what additional benefits can be provided from local government sources. The system as a whole will be explained by your Citizens' Advice Bureau. The broad categories of benefit currently are those set out on the following pages.

Asthma may disable for a time and then diminish; this presents a barrier to claiming some of the benefits, and persistence may be needed to obtain them. Additional help may be obtained from the following:

Welfare Rights Officers at the Town Hall

D.H.S.S., Leaflets Unit, P O Box 21, Stanmore, Middlesex HA7 1AY

Community Health Councils: see local Telephone Directory

Disabled Living Foundation, 380/384 Harrow Road, London W9 2HU (Tel. 01-289 6111)

Disability Alliance, 25 Denmark Street, London WC2H 8NJ (Tel. 01-240 0806)

Mobility Allowance Unit: D.H.S.S., Warbreck Hill, Blackpool, Lancs FY2 0UZ (Tel. 0253 856123)

Attendance Allowance Unit: D.H.S.S., Norcross, Blackpool, Lancs FY5 3TA (Tel. 0253 856123)

National Association for the Welfare of Children in Hospital, Argyle House, 29–31 Euston Road, London NW1 2SD (Tel. 01-833 2041)

The new D.H.S.S. leaflet H.B.5, entitled 'Social Security, a Guide to Non-Contributory Benefits', will be found especially helpful.

D.H.S.S. Benefit	Qualification	National Insurance Leaflet Number
Statutory Sick Pay	up to 8 weeks' sickness; paid by employer	
Invalidity Benefit	a pension paid after 28 weeks' sickness	
Severe Disablement Allowance	for people of working age with 80% disablement	NI.252
Mobility Allowance	unable to walk out of doors for at least a year	NI.211
Motability Allowance	the above, used to lease a car	
Attendance Allowance	help needed with eating, cleaning, dressing, etc.	NI.205
Invalid Care Allowance	for those looking after invalids and who, as a result, are not able to work	NI.212
Disablement Benefit	illness due to conditions at work which affect all the workers	NI.237
Disablement Benefit	for a Prescribed Industrial Disease such as occupational asthma	

D.H.S.S. Benefit	Qualification
Social Fund Benefit: from the Budget Fund	A loan, repayable over 12 months, for equipment needed because of the illness (for example, a vacuum cleaner to remove dust; special bedding)
Income Support	An asthmatic may benefit if unemployed or sick, according to scales which vary according to circumstances
Help with payment for medicines	An exemption Certificate may be obtained from the D.H.S.S.; take Form P.11 for the doctor to sign

D.H.S.S Benefit	Qualification
Pre-payment certificates	The 'Season Ticket'. Runs for 4 or 12 months. Saves money if you need more than 5 items a month. Form FP.95, obtained from Post Office or chemist, sent to Family Practitioner Committee

Local Authority Social Services	
Miscellaneous	Based on needs rather than means. Varies from one L.A. to another: e.g. bus passes, telephones, adaptation to homes, nurseries, play groups
Housing Benefit	If income falls, due to illness

Chapter Ten

ALTERNATIVE MEDICINE

Changing attitudes to medicine

In Shakespeare's time, illnesses were treated by infusions made from plants as approved by custom or the herbals. Apothecaries existed in the towns; but they did not receive their charter until 1607, shortly before Shakespeare's death. In our own times, the apothecary's remedies are provided by a science-based industry which spends countless millions on research, while herbal remedies are shunned by the orthodox doctors. We do, of course, take infusions of tea and coffee, but these were unknown to the Elizabethans.

It may at first seem that 'scientific' and 'local' medicine have grown far apart. Their differences can however be over-emphasized. Many of the drugs used for treating asthma derive from plants used as remedies in ancient times. A few miles from where I live, the search continues. At the Brompton Hospital, Professor Barry Kay's team is investigating the leaves of the Gingka Biluba tree, used by the Chinese for thousands of years as a remedy for chest disorders.

Some would question whether the procedures of modern science are fundamentally different from those of 'primitive' medicine-men: both proceed by trial and error; both try in ingenious ways to render the toxic elements inactive while keeping their beneficial properties; both depend on the trust and faith of the recipients; both use esoteric language to describe the mysteries of their craft. There is, however, one big difference. Orthodox medicine draws its conclusions from very carefully controlled trials in which the active drug is tested against a placebo (a substance which is inert) not just on a handful of patients but on many. In contrast, the evidence in support of unorthodox medicine tends to take the form of anecdote, stories of individual cases which have not been studied in a strictly scientific way.

Can 'alternative' medicine help asthmatics?

There are at least 130 alternative systems for treating our human ailments and many of these aim to treat respiratory illnesses. Few of the books which describe these remedies provide anything resembling proofs that they are effective. This is not surprising, since many of them were established long before modern science took over our civilization. They survived through the centuries because, for one reason or another, they made people feel better. It is only in the last year or so that a serious scientific study of these disciplines has been initiated, and the conclusions will not become known until the turn of the century. This is in contrast with the vast amount of evidence, from both clinical and laboratory studies, that orthodox treatments do work, especially where severe life-threatening attacks are concerned. So until there is hard scientific evidence that alternative medicine can provide better results it should be used not as alternative but as **complementary** medicine. Seen in this light, alternative procedures often have the approval of conventional practitioners. It is, however, a good idea to consult your orthodox doctor as to the suitability of any system you may wish to try before you undertake a course of treatment.

A non-orthodox consultation may have its advantages. In *Living With Allergies*, Dr John McKenzie has written:

> Alternative therapies are comforting, and a visit to a therapist is generally going to be a pleasant, soothing experience, which is rarely true of visits to hospitals or surgeries ... The emphasis of many alternative therapies is to treat the whole patient on many levels simultaneously, with the final aim of reaching the point where the patient can maintain good health unaided.

Some complementary systems described

Acupuncture

This is a fully developed system of medicine, practised in China for over 3,000 years, which rests on a view of life which supposes that the whole universe is ruled by the interplay of 'Yin' and 'Yang'. These are opposing forces which have to be kept in balance when they operate within the body. If one organ is stimulated, then another will be sedated; and the balance will also be affected by universal forces such as the weather.

To a Western mind, this may at first sound strange and even absurd, until you recall that an illness such as asthma is swayed by shifts in the balance between the sympathetic and the parasympathetic autonomic nervous system; and any asthmatic will assent to the idea that the weather plays an important part in the ups and downs of the illness.

Western medicine does recognize that an organ which is diseased can produce pain at a distance and uses this to help diagnosis; but in Chinese medicine it provides a basis for treatment, which takes place at the surface. The Chinese believe that there is a kind of life force or 'Chi' which flows through channels, which they call 'meridians', beneath the skin. They think that the force can be redirected by stimulating acupuncture points, which lie along these pathways. In modern practice, the stimulation is carried out with long, thin, disposable, stainless-steel needles, a process which has been described as almost painless. The needles are inserted to a depth of between a fraction of an inch and two inches, and sometimes they are rotated between the thumb and forefinger.

These life-force channels have not been identified by Western medicine, but neurologists accept that acupuncture can sometimes produce prolonged relief from pain. One theory is that the pressure points can release the body's own pain-killing substances, the endorphins, which resemble morphine and heroin, and the body's own hormones. Another theory is that acupuncture blocks nervous impulses transmitted from the spinal cord. A third idea is that acupuncture makes use of the body's electrical fields, which can affect every human cell. That the fourteen channels or 'meridians' exist is not doubted by Chinese practitioners. It is possible for electricity to pass through a substance without changing it and to find its own pathway which does not depend on any that we can directly observe. The pathways have been explored by Chinese professors in various ways. One is by percussion, which generates waves that pass along the meridians; another is by electrical impedance, or resistance, at various points; a third is through radioactive tracers; a fourth, the measurement of local temperature. All these investigations point to the same pathways. This still does not explain 'how it works' – but then orthodox medicine does not understand how aspirin works!

This area of speculation is fascinating, but our immediate concern is whether acupuncture can help the asthmatic. To treat asthma the acupuncturist tries to control the 'Chi' through one or more of four meridians: the lung meridian, the bladder meridian, the heart meridian, the colon meridian; and the point of the ear can be used as well. An acute attack, mild or severe, would be treated, and swiftly relieved, by applying the needle to the 'Ding Chuan' point, just below the neck, and to other points which are referred to by a Chinese name or code (for example, 'Feishu' is Bl 13, or the thirteenth point along the bladder meridian). In China, relief from asthmatic spasm is seen as only a preliminary, and the aim is to control the asthma on a permanent basis without the need for any medicines. Any lesser state would be seen as 'crippling'. For establishing control on a longer term, that is, reducing inflammation and hyper-responsiveness, additional points would be used such as 'Lieque' (Lung 7). Hay fever and rhinitis can be eliminated, it is claimed, by adding two more points: 'Yintang' and 'Yingaxiang'. Not many controlled trials have been published. In a recent trial in India using forty-two patients, the best results were achieved with those asthmatics whose asthma was mainly allergic and of comparatively recent onset and where there was no dependence on steroids.

The sceptic may ask how the acupuncture points have been determined in relation to any particular illness. The acupuncturist will reply that they have been established by trial and error, and the evidence has been amassed by the Chinese universities, whose research teams can draw on the results of large numbers of treatments carried out each year, running into millions if all illnesses are considered.

One of the fascinating aspects of acupuncture is that diagnosis depends in part on the taking of pulses along the radial artery below the wrist, not just one pulse but as many as half a dozen where a really skilled Chinese practitioner is concerned. Blood travels along the artery in waves; by taking the pulse at, say, three points along its course, on the underside of the wrist, the character of the waves can be determined. If stronger at one of the three points than at another, the system is seen to be out of balance and will need correcting until the pulses are even. The pattern of these wave rhythms helps determine the diagnosis.

There are about 5,000 acupuncturists in Europe, but only a few hundred in the United Kingdom. The address of an Acupuncture Association which keeps a registry will be found under 'Useful Addresses' beginning on page 212, along with other addresses relating to complementary medicine. As far as asthma is concerned, the patient will attend every week until between five and ten treatments have been carried out. This could be sufficient to establish control without further weekly sessions, but a return visit will be made if the symptoms reappear. Orthodox medicines can be taken, but the aim of treatment is to reduce dependency on them.

Herbal medicine

Many preparations used in orthodox medicine to treat asthma were derived, ultimately, from plants. The difference between orthodox and herbal medicine is that in the orthodox kind the active ingredient has been identified and isolated; in herbal medicine, either the whole plant is used or a part in its entirety. In defence of this non-selective system it is argued that the plants often contain secondary substances which may make the effective ingredient either stronger or safer.

It is one of the principles of herbal remedies that if possible, they should be based on local plants, preferably gathered at an appropriate time of day, because the chemicals in plants change from hour to hour. It follows that many herbalists grow the plants they need in their own gardens. As an example of this principle, there have been reports of asthma being dramatically improved when local unstrained honey has been swallowed, presumably because it has reduced sensitivity to some of the local pollens.

The aim in choosing a remedy is not, as in conventional medicine, to block any of the body's reactions but to treat the patient as a whole and to stimulate the body's own defences. In asthma, however, the treatments are usually anti-spasmodic and are used in conjunction with the orthodox bronchodilators, at least in the early stages. The doses are small – but not homeopathically small – and side effects are rare. Of concern to orthodox doctors are those imported remedies which contain steroids in excessive amounts. The herbs used to treat asthma often have beautiful names, such as celandine, elder flower, fennel, hyssop and valerian.

One of the advantages of herbalism is that the practitioner does not simply prescribe a herbal remedy but takes a very detailed history, in the expectation that the underlying causes can be tackled at source. This history goes back to childhood, and great attention is paid to diet, lifestyle, exercise and breathing technique. As far as diet is concerned, the herbalists distinguish between what they see as acid-forming foods and acid-binding foods. The former include meat, cheese, cereals and nuts and are believed to increase the production of mucus in the airways. The acid-binding foods are thought to diminish mucus; they include fruits, root vegetables, milk, cane sugar, coconut and oysters. Since the turn of the present century, herbalists have advised people to keep separate those foods which need different digestive enzymes, and to take them at different times, broadly distinguishing between proteins (which, they say, leave acid residues) and cereals (which leave alkaline residues). They advise that a natural diet is to be preferred to one which contains chemical additives.

Homeopathy

This is a complete system of medicine which rests on the principle that 'like can cure like': a substance which can produce certain symptoms in a healthy person at a large dose can, in a sick person, relieve those same symptoms when given in a tiny dose. This principle can be illustrated by an example. In the early nineteenth century, a certain Dr Hahnemann noticed that a large extract of Cinchona bark produced symptoms like those of malaria. This suggests that the dilute extract is stimulating the systems in the body which fight disease in much the same way that vaccines are used nowadays in immunization.

What at first seems to defy scientific logic is that the strength or 'potency' of a homeopathic remedy increases as the dilution increases. This dilution can consist of taking a tenth part of a solution of the substance in water or alcohol and by 'succussion' shaking it vigorously with ten parts of the diluent, and so on for as many as thirty dilutions. By the time the thirtieth succussion has been completed there may remain in the solution not a single molecule of the original substance. Homeopathic practitioners sometimes explain this in terms of modern physics, which tells us that it is energy and not mass which lies at the heart of matter and that it is possible for the energy of the diluent to be greatly increased by each successive dilution and for the water or alcohol molecules to be changed. This energy, it is suggested, can stimulate a response at the level of our body cells.

Of greater interest to asthma sufferers is the question, whether any of these remedies can relieve their symptoms. Like herbalists, the homeopathic doctors are interested in the possible triggers for asthma or hay fever; many are also qualified in orthodox medicine and prescribe conventional and homeopathic medicines at the same time. So it may be difficult to decide which of the three approaches contributes most to any improvement. The following case has been described: a girl of four had severe asthma which, over two years, did not respond to any of the inhalers. At the homeopathic clinic, skin tests showed a strong allergic reaction to house dust mite extract. The homeopathic doctor prescribed a homeopathically prepared solution of house dust and, at the same time, persuaded the mother to buy a solid foam mattress with a plastic cover and provide terylene pillows. Subsequently, after one dose of the homeopathic preparation, the symptoms of asthma disappeared and no more medicines of any kind were needed.

A third principle of homeopathy, which may puzzle anyone who believes (as I do) that asthma is not an illness of nervous origin, is that the choice of homeopathic remedy is determined not only by the illness but also by the type of personality or 'constitution' that is being treated. Rather in the same way that the ancient Greeks identified people as having 'humours' which made them phlegmatic, choleric, melancholic or sanguine in temperament, so the homeopathist decides whether the patient is independent or gregarious, tidy or untidy, anxious or confident; the type of asthma is also considered. Thus a patient who complains of night asthma and who has a restless and anxious spirit is treated with Arsenicum. Calmer patients with night asthma are more likely to respond to Ipecac. If the patient is sweet-tempered and affectionate and dislikes stuffy rooms, then Pulsatilla is tried. Ipacac is preferred if there is a copious production of phlegm, whereas if the asthma is dry or there is pronounced wheezing, then the therapist is likely to prescribe Spongia or Bryonia. If the asthma is easily provoked by emotion, especially anger, then Chamomilla is considered, and this is also used in children whose asthma makes them irritable.

This view – that asthma is linked to types of personality – is not generally shared by psychiatrists. The opposite view – that asthma may profoundly affect the personality – is easy to accept and this does perhaps support the notion that a study of the personality can throw some light on the severity of the illness.

Homeopathy is practised by some 300 medically trained doctors in the United Kingdom, who are also qualified in orthodox medicine and use both systems in conjunction. The homeopathic medicines are available under the National Health Service and there are six homeopathic hospitals within the service. The Faculty of Homeopathy is legally recognized; and both the present Queen and her father, George VI, have been patrons of the Royal London Homeopathic Hospital.

Treatment is given in the smallest doses that will bring relief. In an attack of asthma they will be given every ten minutes, then every fifteen minutes, with an increasing interval of time until a dose given once every twenty-four hours is reached. Constitutional remedies may need to be taken only as a single dose. Quite startling changes may be experienced, but these are not toxic effects and the medicines can be regarded as safe, cheap, easy to take, taste-free and capable of being stored for long periods.

As with the other complementary medicines, an official Commission is investigating the claims of homeopathy and by 1999 will decide whether these remedies can continue to be prescribed on the National Health Service.

Hypnosis

The aim in hypnosis is to increase a patient's acceptance of the treatment proposed and to achieve a greater degree of relaxation before an attack. The patient can be persuaded, under hypnosis, that the autonomic system will function normally and not (as in asthma) swing too far towards the parasympathetic side of the autonomic pendulum. Hypnosis goes back to the Greeks and the Druids, but its fame in Europe dates from the 1760s when Franz Mesmer gave dramatic and sometimes hilarious demonstrations of his powers.

The way hypnotism works is as follows: the hypnotist persuades the subject to fix the eyes on an image such as a revolving wheel. The eye-muscles become fatigued and the eyes close. The therapist then talks in a slow monotonous voice and suggests that the patient relax until a trance-like hypnotic state, somewhere between sleeping and waking, is achieved. Most people can be hypnotized and reach the stage of believing that what they are told will happen, provided that this is not at variance with their personal code of conduct.

Hypnosis will not relieve an attack already under way, but there have been cases in which it has helped asthmatics to achieve a state of calm relaxation when the wheezes first appear and so avoid a serious attack. Patients can be taught how to put themselves into a trance and practise 'auto-hypnosis' when they feel an attack coming on. Hypnosis can also help smokers to give up their habit. It is essential to use the services of a therapist who is also trained in orthodox medicine; a list of such practitioners can be obtained from the British Society of Medical and Dental Hypnosis (see 'Useful Addresses', page 212).

Manipulative therapies

Osteopaths remind us that, in the long history of evolution, Man has only recently walked on two feet with an upright posture. We put loads on the discs between our vertebrae which they were not originally designed to bear and, in our upright state, the organs hang down in an abnormal way. This can, under strain, set up stresses at the point where muscles attach to bones, and these can be painful if the affected area is close to a nerve. Osteopathy can free the tissue from strain and permit a better flow of blood not only to the nearby organs but also to more distant parts of the body.

This has some relevance to asthma, because the nerve supply to the lungs comes through the spinal cord and manipulation can remove abnormal strains that bear upon this nervous pathway. The osteopaths also believe, as do physiotherapists, that asthmatics tend to breathe using the muscles of the chest rather than the diaphragm, and also to breathe through the mouth. This, as we have already seen, can contribute to the asthmatic response, and it can be corrected. Osteopaths are also concerned with the patient's environment and way of life as a contributing factor.

Chiropracters are concerned more narrowly with the spine and posture. Qualified osteopaths and chiropracters, those who are registered by their associations, have undergone a rigorous training and know much more about joints than orthodox doctors in general practice. It is at least questionable, so far as the lungs are concerned, whether they have much to contribute in the way of additional insights beyond those of orthodox medicine. It is worth adding that anyone can set up, without training, as a manipulative therapist; only a registered practitioner should be consulted.

Reflexology

This is a very old system, which in ancient China was used in conjunction with acupuncture. The principle is that, by deeply massaging certain parts of the body, beneficial effects are produced elsewhere. In the West, practitioners concentrate on the feet, not in the way chiropodists do, but because it is believed that very specific parts of the feet relate, in some mysterious way, to distant parts of the body, including the lungs. As the therapist gently strokes the surface, pain is felt in the 'sensitive area' and this, together with a crystalline feeling to the touch, shows where the deep massage should take place. Deep massage is carried out with the edge of the finger or thumb, in a circular motion. Orthodox medicine cannot detect any nervous pathways which might connect the feet with the internal organs in this very specific way, but the system can claim successes, including relief from asthma. The foot is very well represented in the brain and this may be a clue to the route by which the stimulus is transmitted.

Yoga

Yoga is now practised by many people in the West as a means of achieving both suppleness and relaxation and is a very old discipline, stretching back at least to 3000 B.C. Over the years many different forms have developed, often centred on a guru (one who dispels darkness). The aim has been to explore all the bodily functions and use correct breathing and posture to prevent or cure disease.

Each posture consists of a movement of the body, a mental state and a control of breathing. Breathing is especially important. Slow and controlled breathing, when it has been achieved, creates a state of calmness and is conducive to meditation. Highly disciplined teachers can reduce their breathing rate to two breaths a minute or raise it to sixty times that rate, at will.

Can yoga help people with asthma? A study has been reported in the *British Medical Journal* in which a sizeable number of asthmatics were treated with yoga in addition to conventional medicine. Compared with the controls (people who had only the medicines) the asthmatics had fewer symptoms and needed fewer drugs. The authors of this report looked for a reason and wondered whether yoga may have dampened the 'parasympathetic response', which causes a narrowing of the airways. What can be said with certainty is that yoga is the most profound way in which to learn relaxation.

Surprisingly, there is no register of qualified practitioners, but some local authorities include yoga classes in the programmes of their adult institutes.

Chapter Eleven

THE WORK OF THE ASTHMA SOCIETY

A problem shared is generally reckoned to be a problem halved. The Asthma Society currently has 160 branches, large and small, spread around the kingdom; it exists to help asthmatics and their parents share the experience of coping with the illness. As one member told me 'I wish I had known about these activities when my daughter first had asthma: I had to learn the hard way how to cope.'

The branches hold meetings which are open to the public and are addressed by specialists. They distribute leaflets on varied aspects of the illness, and *Asthma News*, which has a circulation of around 40,000 copies, covers both medical topics and branch news. Branches lend members video and audio tapes, made by doctors for the pharmaceutical companies.

Some branches equip doctors with nebulizers, and peak flow meters can be obtained from the Head Office at cost price. Some branches organize Swim Groups and others provide dry-land exercises. Activity holidays are arranged for asthmatic children, who obtain thereby a great increase in self-confidence. In addition to that, the branches put on events which raise money for the Asthma Research Council. This supports fundamental research into asthma in hospitals around the country, including two professorial chairs.

The Asthma Society Training Centre

This was set up in February 1987 to provide training, over a three-day course, for nurses and health visitors who want to learn more about practical management of the illness. It is financed in part by the Asthma Society and its location at Stratford-upon-Avon could not be more pleasant. Emphasis is laid on case-studies, involving real patients; those attending find that their insight into asthma is greatly enhanced.

Chapter Twelve

THE QUESTIONS PEOPLE ASK – AND WHERE TO FIND THE ANSWERS

Among the many questions people ask about asthma, there are some that crop up with great frequency. The cross-references following the questions are to the page numbers of this book where the answers will be found.

Symptoms and signs

'How do I know it is asthma and not bronchitis?'
    Page 54.

'Should I have a skin prick test?'
    Page 40.

'Is asthma a dangerous illness?'
    Page 7.

'When should I call the doctor?'
    Pages 113, 134.

Causes

'Are asthma and hay fever inherited?'
    Pages 28, 123.

'Are asthmatics people who are unduly nervous?'
    Page 175.

'Why is asthma often worse at night?'
    Page 56.

'Can colds cause symptoms of asthma?'
    Page 54.

'Are asthma and hay fever always due to allergy?'
  Pages 6, 158.

'Can changes in the weather affect asthma and hay fever?'
  Page 47.

Precautions

'Should I give up smoking?'
  Page 50.

'Should I try to eliminate dust from the bedroom?'
  Page 36.

'Do we have to get rid of the pets?'
  Page 38.

'My asthmatic son loves games; should I let him take part?'
  Page 139.

'If we move somewhere else, will the asthma improve?'
  Page 127.

Worries about medicines

'If they are taken day after day, will the effects wear off?'
  Page 62.

'Can I become addicted to the medicines?'
  Page 63.

'If I take more than one medicine, will this increase the side effects?'
  Page 63.

'Do I have to go on taking the medicines even though I have no symptoms?'
  Page 73.

'If the attack gets worse, should I increase the dosage?'
  Page 62.

'How do I know whether my child is using the inhaler correctly?'
  Page 85

'My neighbour's friend has been advised to use a nebulizer. Should I have one too?'
Page 91.

No one understands

'I am not sure my doctor understands my asthma. What should I do?'
Page 179.

'The teachers at school will not let my child use his inhaler when needed. What should I do?'
Page 137.

What about the future?

'Will my child grow out of asthma?'
Page 127.

'Should I have another child?'
Page 124.

A. *The secret life of cells*

The allergic response proceeds in this way:

1 The pollen grain (i.e. the antigen) enters the airways and
2 latches on to a **mast cell**. It is able to do this because:

• the mast cell has escaped from its usual home under the cell linings

• the antigen meets an antibody attached to the mast cell which is adapted to receive it (and no other kind of antigen)

3 Many asthmatics have leaky mast cells which, in response to the hook-up described above, burst open and release the granules within.

4 These contain **mediators**, such as histamine, which can cause a response in the cells which occupy the airways:

• the linings become inflamed

• they secrete mucus

• they also become leaky

5 Gaps now appearing in the weakened tissue cells allow pollen grains to pass through them. Grains may meet mast cells lying under the tissues and latch on to their antibodies, releasing more mediators and causing a build-up of inflammation.

6 As if this were not enough, it is also possible that chemicals released by the inflamed and weakened tissue cells will set off a nervous response (similar to the cough reflex) in the muscles surrounding the air passages, causing them to go into spasm.

7 If the patient is anxious or excited, then these neural messages may be reinforced.

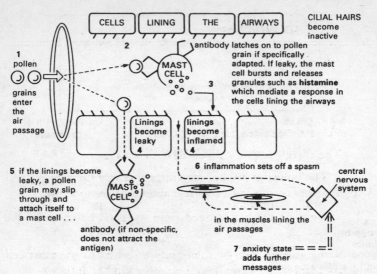

Fig 22 (See also Fig 23 on page 202)

B. What the doctor needs to know

In order to make a correct diagnosis and decide upon a course of treatment, the doctor needs to learn a good deal about the patient's symptoms and lifestyle, as well as making any necessary tests. The tests may include a measurement of peak flow, preferably taken over a week; also a reversibility test to show whether peak flow improves after a bronchodilator has been used. A measurement of height will be needed to relate peak flow to the predicted levels for the age and sex of the patient.

None of this need be in any way alarming, and it is a good plan to turn up at the first consultation with the answers ready to the kind of questions that may be asked:

• the year in which the symptoms started

• any history in the family of asthma, eczema, hay fever or urticaria

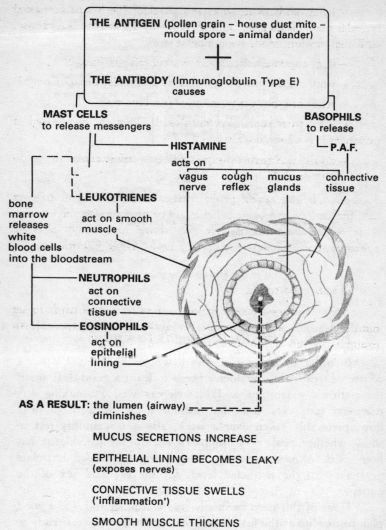

THE ANTIGEN (pollen grain – house dust mite –
mould spore – animal dander)

+

THE ANTIBODY (Immunoglobulin Type E)
causes

MAST CELLS
to release messengers

BASOPHILS
to release

HISTAMINE
acts on

P.A.F.

vagus   cough   mucus   connective
nerve   reflex   glands   tissue

bone
marrow
releases
white
blood cells
into the bloodstream

LEUKOTRIENES
act on smooth
muscle

NEUTROPHILS
act on
connective
tissue

EOSINOPHILS
act on
epithelial
lining

AS A RESULT: the lumen (airway)
diminishes

MUCUS SECRETIONS INCREASE

EPITHELIAL LINING BECOMES LEAKY
(exposes nerves)

CONNECTIVE TISSUE SWELLS
('inflammation')

SMOOTH MUSCLE THICKENS

Fig 23. Full Allergic Response (inflammation and secretion, as well as muscle spasm)

• what tends to provoke the attacks? The list to be ticked includes seasonal factors, animals, house dust, head colds, exercise, cold air, emotion, food, something at work

• does anyone in the family smoke? Do you smoke?

• what are the present symptoms? (Mucus? Wheeze? Cough?)

• when are the symptoms most troublesome?

• what treatments have been used? What are being used at present? How many times a day?

• do the treatments disappear shortly after treatment, or do they fail to respond?

An allergist would probe further into the kind of triggers that the patient or parent believes are responsible for the attacks. It is worth mentioning that the above list would also be appropriate to an investigation by an unorthodox practitioner.

Treatment cards

Some doctors are now making use of treatment cards to set out the doses needed as a routine and if the asthma gets worse. An example is given on the next page.

TREATMENT TO BE TAKEN REGULARLY

Name	Dose: (No. of puffs or tablets)	No. of doses daily

Don't forget your regular treatment.

RELIEF TREATMENT IF YOUR ASTHMA GETS WORSE

For sudden chest tightness, wheeze or breathlessness take:

Name:	Dose and how taken:
1.	
2.	
3.	

if no relief or quickly worse:

●   repeat relief treatment

●   also take ....tablets of prednisolone*

And at the same time:

●   Contact your GP*

●   or dial 999 for an ambulance*

●   or go to.................Hospital

  * complete/delete as necessary

Keep your inhalers handy at all times

IF YOU USE A PEAK FLOW METER FOLLOW THESE GUIDELINES

Expected Peak Flow _____ l/min

Best Peak Flow _____ l/min

If your Peak Expiratory Flow (PEF) suddenly falls below _____ use relief treatment in the order listed.

If no relief or quickly worse again or if PEF at any time below _____ take emergency action listed opposite.

If your morning PEF is regularly below _____ or you are waking at night with your asthma, *see your doctor.*

You can obtain a Peak Flow Meter from the Asthma Society or through your doctor.

Fig 24. Example of a Treatment Card which is now available to be used by doctors in the management of asthma, designed to save the patient from taking notes of what is prescribed. (Courtesy of the Asthma Society)

C. A brief guide to the medicines

Group A: *The bronchodilators: the relievers*

	adrenaline derivatives	caffeine derivatives	atropine derivative
use	to relieve wheeze and shortage of breath, once started	they also relax the airways, by a different route	the same action, by a third route, especially useful in infants
form	mostly taken by inhalation; syrups and slow-release tablets also available	usually taken as a slow-relcase tablet	taken by inhalation
side effects	a tremor known popularly as 'the shakes'	non-selective bronchodilators which stimulate the heart and affect all the body tissues	no side effects at the normal dose
brand names	Berotec Bricanyl Pulmadil Ventolin Ventodisks	Choledyl Nuelin SA Phyllocontin Slo-Phyllin Uniphyllin	Atrovent (Duovent)

At any one time only one drug is used from each sub-group, but drugs from the sub-groups are sometimes combined, for example Ventolin and Atrovent.

Colour of inhalers: blue or grey.

Group B: *The preventers*

	anti-inflammatory steroids	Nedocromil	anti-allergic sodium cromoglycate
use	for prevention, not for relieving attacks, so must be taken at least twice a day every day if inhaled	for prevention only	for prevention only, and especially useful in children
form	taken by inhalation and in small tablet doses	taken by inhalation	taken by inhalation
side effects	numerous side effects: at doses higher than those prescribed for prevention	no significant side effects	no significant side effects
brand names	Becodisks Becotide Becloforte Pulmicort Prednisolone	Tilade	Intal

The preventers are usually taken in conjunction with one of the relieving drugs; drugs from within the steroid sub-group can be combined (e.g. inhaled and tablet steroid) and so are drugs from different sub-groups (e.g. Tilade and Becotide).

Colour of inhalers: beige, brown and red.

Group C: *Life-savers in an acute attack*

	bronchodilators	steroids
form	nebulized, or given by injection	taken as tablets, in a high dose, or given by injection

They are often used in combination, since they act by different routes.

D. How doses compare when taken in different ways

(Ventolin is given as an example)

form	size of dose per tablet or puff or nebule	doses which are generally recommended			
		age	dose	times a day	maximum in 24 hours
('oral route')					
tablet	2 mg. or 4 mg.	infant	nil		
		2–6 years	1–2 mg.		
syrup		6–12 years	2 mg.	3 or 4	
		adult	2–4 mg.	up to 4	16 mg.
slow-release tablet*	8 mg.	child	nil		
		adult	1	up to 2	16 mg.
metered-dose aerosol inhaler (as used for regular treatment)	100 µg.	child	½ adult		
		adult	up to 2 puffs	4-hourly	
inhaled powder**	200 µg.	child	½ adult		
		adult	up to 2 puffs	4-hourly	
nebulizer	2.5–5 mg.	adult	1–2 nebules	4-hourly	20 mg.
injection	500 mg.	(dose relates to body weight)		4-hourly	
(subcutaneous or intramuscular)					

* Volmax   ** Rotacaps

The size of the doses discharged may be compared in the following chart:

10 mg. by nebulizer	=	100 times
4 mg. by oral tablet	=	40 times
400 µg. by Rotacap	=	4 times

the amount discharged by inhaler (100 µg.)

1,000 micrograms (µg.) = 1 milligram (mg.)

E. The forms in which the drugs are available (*the list is not exhaustive*)

Generic name	Brand	Made by	RELIEVERS Inhalers			Nebulizer	Swallowed Syrup	Tablets
			Aerosol	Spacer	Dry Powders			
Bronchodilators								
salbutamol	Ventolin	A.H.	*	Volumatic	Rotahaler	*	*	slow-release
(+ steroid)	Ventodisks	A.H.			Diskhaler			Spandet
	Ventide	A.H.	*					*
	Salbulin	3M Riker	*					
	Aerolin	3M Riker	Auto					
	Volmax	D.F.						Volmax
terbutaline	Bricanyl	Astra	*	Nebuhaler	Turbohaler	*	*	*
orciprenaline	Alupent	Boehr.	*				*	*
fenoterol	Berotec	Boehr.	*			*		
(+ ipratropium)	Duovent	Boehr.						
reproterol	Bronchodil	Degasser	*			*		*
rimiterol	Pulmadil	3M Riker	*					
	Pulmadil	3M Riker	Auto					
aminophylline	Phyllocontin	Napp						*
theophylline	Nuelin S.A.	3M Riker					*	SR
	Slo-Phyllin	Lipa						capsules
	Theograd	Abbott						*
	Theo-Dur	Astra						*
	Uniphyllin	Napp						*
ipratropium	Atrovent	Boehr.	*			*		

A.H. Allen & Hanbury   D.F. Duncan Flockhart   Boehr. Boehringer

Generic name	Brand	Made by	PREVENTERS Inhalers Aerosol	Spacer	Dry Powders	Nebulizer	Swallowed Syrup	Tablets
Anti-allergic								
ketotifen	Zaditen						*	*
sodium cromoglycate	Intal	Fisons	*		Spinhaler	*		
(+ isoprenalene)	Intal Co.	Fisons			Spinhaler			
Anti-Inflammatory (steroids)								
beclomethasone diproprionate	Becotide	A.H.	50/100	Volumatic	Rotahaler	*		
	Becodisks	A.H.			Diskhaler			
	Becloforte	A.H.		Volumatic				
budesonide	Pulmicort	Astra	50	Nebuhaler				
			200	Nebuhaler				
betamethasone valerate	Bextasol	Glaxo	*					
hydrocortisone	Hydrocortistab	Boots						*
	Hydrocortone	M.S.D.						*
prednisone	Prednesol	Glaxo						*
	Deltacortril	Pfizer						*
	Deltastab	Boots						*
	Precortisyl	Roussel						*
methyl-prednisolone	Medrone	Upjohn						*
Anti-inflammatory (others)								
nedocromil	Tilade	Fisons	*					

A.H. Allen & Hanbury. M.S.D. Merck, Sharp & Dohme.

Radioactive tracers have been used to discover how much drug is delivered to the breathing tubes, and how much is lost on the way. When a metered-dose aerosol inhaler is used, 8–10% reaches the target; a collapsible spacer puts this up to about 17%; a Nebuhaler achieves about 30% efficiency and a nebulizer, because very small particles are achieved, is still more efficient. The caffeine derivatives can be absorbed through the 'buccal route' under the tongue, as well as being swallowed, so an efficient delivery is essential when the asthma is at all severe to make sure that as much as possible ends up in the breathing tubes.

F. Will they ever find a cure for asthma?

This question is often asked by asthmatics and their families. If asthma is seen to be an inappropriate response to triggers, a response passed in various ways from one generation to another, research into the illness can follow four different pathways. The scientists can look at the genes which are handed down through families; they can study the triggers present in the environment; they can study in microscopic detail the lungs' response to these stimuli; and they can devise and test drugs which are designed to block this response.

In the last few years advances have been made on all four fronts. As we have seen, geneticists have discovered where, on the long DNA molecule, the faulty genes can be found and they are throwing light on exactly what responses can be transmitted through the generations. Cell biologists are now able, with very sensitive equipment, to show how the whole complicated mechanism of asthma is fired into action.

The environment is being studied intensively both in very small communities and in very large ones. By taking a village with a stable population and studying all the families over a number of years, it is possible to show in what way the asthmatic families differ from the others in matters such as diet, smoking and exposure to allergens. Scientists are also looking at much larger groups of people to see if dietary factors play a part on a large scale. Is the absence of asthma in Eskimos, they are asking, due to their reliance on fish and high intake of fish oil? Is there a link in Europe as a whole between varying levels of salt intake and the varying levels in the severity of asthma in different parts of the continent?

All this work provides pointers for the scientists in the pharmaceutical industry in their search for drugs which can block the asthmatic response at various stages. They are not only working with chemical compounds which are already known but are looking afresh at remedies derived from plants and used for centuries in 'primitive' medicine. The living plants are themselves being rescued from the danger of extinction.

There is an air of expectancy these days in the scientific community. Advances in understanding crowd in upon them so that in 1987 the Chairman of the Asthma Research Council was moved to write in her Annual Report, 'for the first time the chances of finding a cure for asthma appear to be real'.

USEFUL ADDRESSES

Self-help Societies

Asthma Society and Friends of the Asthma Research Council
300 Upper Street, London N1 2XX (Tel. 01-226 2260)
(see page 195 for a description of the Society's activities)

Asthma Society Training Centre
22 Scholars' Lane, Stratford-upon-Avon, Warwickshire
CV37 6HE
(Tel. 0789 292201 or 296974)

The Lung Foundation
Kingsmead House, 250 King's Road, SW3 5UE (Tel. 01-376 5735)
This concerns itself with all respiratory illnesses.

Chest, Heart and Stroke Association
Tavistock House North, Tavistock Square, London WC1H
9JE (Tel. 01-387 3012)
Provides useful booklets and a magazine, *Hope*, in which
people describe how they have learnt to cope with their dis-
abilities.

National Eczema Society
Tavistock House North, Tavistock Square, London WC1H
9SR (Tel. 01-388 4097)

Action Against Allergy
43 The Downs, London SW20 8HG (Tel. 01-947 5082)

Asthma Society of Ireland
24 Anglesea Street, Dublin 2 (Tel. 01-716551)

Asthma Care Association of America
PO Box 568, Spring Valley Road, Ossining, NY 10562 (Tel. 914 762 1941)

Complementary Medicine

Institute of Complementary Medicine
21 Portland Place, London W1N 3AF (Tel. 01-636 9543)

British Holistic Medical Association
179 Gloucester Place, London NW1 6DX (Tel. 01-262 5299)

British Acupuncture Association and Register
34 Alderney Street, London SW1V 4EU (Tel. 01-834 1012)

National Institute of Medical Herbalists
41 Hatherly Road, Winchester, Hampshire SO22 6RR
Send s.a.e. for list of practitioners and leaflets.

British Homeopathic Association
27A Devonshire Street, London W1N 1RJ (Tel. 01-935 2163)
They can supply a list of homeopathic doctors and many publications.

British Society of Medical and Dental Hypnosis
42 Links Road, Ashtead, Surrey KT21 2HJ (Tel. 03722 73522)
Can supply a list of medically qualified practitioners: send s.a.e.

General Council and Register of Osteopaths Ltd
1–4 Suffolk Street, London SW1Y 4HG (Tel. 01-839 2060)

General Health Education

Health Education Authority
78 New Oxford Street, London WC1H 9TX (Tel. 01-631 0930)
Their booklet on cutting out smoking, 'A Smoker's Guide To Giving Up', is recommended.

Nutrition Advisory Service
Safeway Food Stores Ltd, Aylesford, Kent ME20 7A1
Useful free booklets on food additives.

A.S.H.
5-11 Mortimer Street, London W1N 7RH (Tel. 01-637 9843)

Medical Equipment etc.

Clement Clarke International Ltd
15 Wigmore Street, London W1H 9LA (Tel. 01-580 8053)
Suppliers of peak flow meters.

Vitalograph Ltd
Maids Moreton House, Buckingham MK18 1SW (Tel. 0280 813691
Also suppliers of peak flow meters.

Medic-Alert Foundation
11 Clifton Terrace, London N4 3JP (Tel. 01-263 8596)
Can supply a Medic-Alert steroid bracelet.

Bubbleheads
Made and sold by Mr R. H. Hincliffe, 10 Bridge Street,
Pershore, Worcester WR10 1AT (Tel. 0386 556292).

Medic-Aid Ltd
Hook Lane, Pagham, Sussex PO21 3PP (Tel. 0423 267321)
Suppliers of nebulizers, compressors and masks.

Medix Ltd
Medix House, Main Street, Catthorpe, Lutterworth, Leics
LE17 6DB (Tel. 0788 860366)
Suppliers of lightweight nebulizing equipment.

Dunlopillo U.K.
Pannal, Harrogate, North Yorks HG3 1JL.
Manufacturers of latex foam mattresses.

Medivac (Taylormade Products) Ltd
20 Bridge Green, Prestbury, Macclesfield, Cheshire SK10
4HR (Tel. 0625 827922)

Suppliers of vacuum cleaners with non-escape filtration and dust removal monitors.

Vorwerk (UK) Ltd
Unit A, Toutley Road, Wokingham, Berks RG1 1JU (Tel. 0734 794878)
Suppliers of 2-motor-system vacuum cleaners with non-escape filtration and variable heads.

FURTHER READING AND SPECIAL ACKNOWLEDGEMENTS

Chapter One · Living with Asthma

I have found it helpful to read various approaches to the subject; one of the most readable introductions, beautifully illustrated, is: *Asthma and Hay Fever* by Dr Allan Knight (Martin Dunitz, 1981). Now a little out of date, but Dr Knight understands the family's concerns. Available from Book Point, Block 39, Milton Trading Estate, nr Abingdon, Oxon.

Page 9: Is asthma a modern illness? I wish I had space to quote more from Dr Sakula's fascinating paper 'A History of Asthma', published by the *Journal of the Royal College of Physicians of London* (Vol. 22, No. 1, Jan. 1988). This traces the history of treatments from earliest times.

Page 10: Are remote rural people free from asthma? This is discussed more fully on pages 113–22 of *Asthma the Facts* by Drs Lane and Storr (Oxford University Press, 2nd edition, 1987). This is a classic of medical literature, written for lay people and doctors alike, a gold mine of information on asthma which will repay reading several times.

Page 11: 'Why do I have asthma?' The quotation is taken from a slim paperback which slips easily into the pocket but is voluminous in the mind: *Adult Asthma* by Professor T. J. H. Clark (Churchill Livingstone, 1984).

An even slimmer volume, just 30 pages long, attractively written but with unsympathetic illustrations, has an equally broad approach: *Life With Asthma* by Dr Wykeham Balme (a Family Doctor booklet published by the British Medical Association, 1986).

I have also derived nourishment from *The A.B.C. of Asthma* by Dr John Rees (B.M.J. Publications, 1984) and from *A Practical Approach to Asthma* by Drs Pawels and Snashall (C.B.A. Services, 1986).

Page 21: Pollen grains and mast cells. The diagram has been derived from *Food Allergy* (Edsall publications), cited in Chapter Seven.

Chapter Two · Which Triggers Cause Asthma?

Page 37: Dust that builds on dust. The diagram has been adapted from another slim booklet: *Asthma in Childhood* by Professor A. D. Milner (Churchill Livingstone, 1984).

Page 47: Getting excited or upset. This is treated more fully in Lane and Storr (see above); in the first chapter, Dr Storr gives a moving account of what it is like to have a severe attack.

Page 47: The mysterious effect of the atmosphere. Dr Jon Ayres's account of the Birmingham thunderstorm was reported in *Asthma News*, December 1987.

Chapter Three · Managing Asthma with Medicines

Page 69: Caffeine derivatives. A recent account of the role of the theophyllines has been given in *Asthma News*, March 1988, by Dr John Harvey.

Page 77: Sodium cromoglycate. A history of the discovery of Intal has been written by Dr John Suschitzky and published in *Chem. Britain* (21 (6):554, 1985).

Page 83: A closer look at inhalers. I am indebted to the pharmaceutical companies for permission to reproduce or adapt drawings published by them, especially to Messrs Allen & Hanbury and Fisons.

Chapter Four · Adjusting Treatment to Suit the Illness

Page 101: The charts have been taken from *Peak Expiratory Flow Meter Measurement in the Management of Asthma*, an excellent booklet devised by Allen & Hanbury for general practitioners, in 1986.

Page 104: How does the doctor choose the treatments? The ideas which underlie this section have been derived from the course for nurses run by the Asthma Society's Training Centre at Stratford-upon-Avon.

Page 110: What you should do if things go wrong. This very useful summary has been taken from a booklet by Dr Douglas Jenkinson, for use by his patients in a trial supported by Allen & Hanbury, with their permission.

Page 117: Peak flow readings can offer guidance. The charts used in this section have been based, with permission, on cards supplied by Fisons Limited to general practitioners to give to their patients. The way in which peak flow readings can guide practitioners has been developed in: *Asthma: the Management in General Practice* by Dr Ian Gregg (Update Publications, 1985).

Page 119: Posture during an attack. The illustrations are based on drawings in a leaflet devised by the physiotherapy department of the Brompton Hospital, London.

Chapter Five · Living with an Asthmatic Child

The best short introduction to this very important topic is *Childhood Asthma* by Professor Nevill Buchanan (Judy Piatkus, London, 1987). It also includes (rare among medical literature) cartoons which are both humorous and sympathetic; it comes from Australia, a country with a very high incidence of asthma.

Other useful booklets include: *Your Child and Asthma* by

Drs Wilson and Pearl, (Astra Pharmaceuticals, Kings Langley, Herts). This has sixteen pages and is well illustrated in full colour, so as to be of interest to older children as well as to parents. *Asthma in Childhood*, already cited, is packed with accessible information in a small format.

I have also found helpful a booklet published by the Nottingham City Hospital, *Coping with Asthma, a Guide for Parents*, in which Mrs Marguerite Howard asks the questions and Dr Joan Hiller provides the answers.

General practitioners can obtain an up-to-date summary of current thinking from a recent monograph: *Asthma in Childhood* by Dr Michael Silverman (Current Medical Literature Ltd, 1985).

I have revised the section on 'Managing asthma in infants' in the light of a talk given to the Asthma Society's Conference in October 1988 by Dr Chris O'Callaghan.

Chapter Six · Living with Adult Asthma

This has received less attention as a separate subject than childhood asthma. Professor Clark's useful booklet, *Adult Asthma*, has already been cited. So has Drs Lane and Storr's *Asthma the Facts*, which deals with adult asthma on pages 95–9 in the 2nd edition.

Page 144: Asthma which is severe and persistent. This useful chart has been adapted from Dr A. J. Wollcock's paper in the *European Journal of Respiratory Diseases* (Vol. 69, 1986), reproduced here with the permission of the publishers.

Page 148: Asthma related to work. The paint sprayer's tale was described by Dr Tony Pickering at the 1987 National Conference of the Asthma Society and reported in *Asthma News*.

Chapter Seven · Living with Food Allergy

An introduction to this subject can be found in *Living with Allergies* by Dr John McKenzie (Penguin, 1987).

My sources have included: *Food Allergy* (Edsall Summary for Health Professionals No. 2, Edsall of London) and 'Food Intolerance and Food Aversion', a Joint Report of the Royal College of Physicians and the British Nutrition Foundation, *Journal of R.C.P. of London* (April 1984).

Chapter Eight · Living with Hay Fever

Books on asthma tend to pay rather little attention to hay fever, a notable exception being *Asthma and Hay Fever*, cited above, under Chapter One. I have drawn my material largely from excellent talks given to the West London Branch of the Asthma Society by Drs Bill Frankland, Robert Davies and Derek Williams. *Hay Fever: No Need To Suffer* by Colin Johnson and Arabella Melville (Corgi Books) is good on ways of avoiding the triggers but out-of-date in relation to medical treatment.

Chapter Nine · The Human Response

Physicians concentrate on physical causes and on medical treatments, and asthma has not received much attention from psychiatrists. This means that the most distressing aspect of asthma and severe hay fever, the way these illnesses interfere with ordinary relationships, remains largely unexplored in print.

In 1966 Dr Aaron Lask wrote, in *Asthma: Attitude and Milieu* (Tavistock), about psychological factors in asthma. In 1970 Drs Zealley, Aitken and Rosenthal published a paper in the *Proceedings* of the Royal Society of Medicine (Vol. 64) in which they concluded a 'psychophysiological investigation' into asthmatic patients with the view that asthmatics are no more and no less neurotic than the rest of the population. In 1983 Dr Aas reported to a symposium in Oslo the view of his Children's Asthma and Allergy Clinic that play, carefully adjusted, is essential for children with severe asthma and providing it calls for an imaginative insight into what is possible. In *Asthma News* (No. 14, 1987) the way asthma affects family relationships was explored by Dr Bryan Lask.

Readers are recommended to turn to *Asthma the Facts*, already cited, for Dr Anthony Storr's introduction, 'Asthma as a Personal Experience', which also touches on the psychology of asthma. In the same book Dr Donald Lane examines the relationship between emotion and asthma.

In *Help Me, Mummy, I Can't Breathe* (Souvenir Press, 1987) Susan Sutherland has written a dramatic account of the ups and downs of life with an asthmatic child.

Chapter Ten · *Alternative Medicine*

An excellent general introduction to this subject, in which thirty-two systems are described, has a few references to asthma and hay fever: *Alternative Medicine* by Dr Andrew Stanway (Penguin, 1986). Penguin also publish *Homeopathy for Everyone* and *Acupuncture and Chiropractic* in the same series.

The various societies whose addresses are given on page 213 of this book will be able to suggest additional reading material and Dr Stanway gives a full reading-list in his book.

In June 1988, a now famous article appeared in the prestigious journal *Nature*, in which a French team claimed to have demonstrated that a homeopathic solution could change other substances in contact with it. In the following month, a team investigating the methods used threw doubt on their validity, but in an inconclusive manner.

INDEX

Technical terms are defined when they first appear